Advance praise for *Applied Cognitive Behavioral Therapy in Schools*

"*Applied Cognitive Behavior Therapy in Schools* fills a critical gap in our training of mental health and special education professionals who work in our nation's schools. By blending the current knowledge and practice of CBT with introductions to school infrastructure and policy, the editors and assembled experts provide newcomers to the field with the critical knowledge needed to select and implement state-of-the-art CBT practices in their own schools."

—**Garret D. Evans**, PsyD, Director,
Florida Consortium for Child and Adolescent Behavioral Health

"The availability of pragmatic tools to assist in the application of skills remains a critical yet often overlooked component of effective training and service delivery. *Applied Cognitive Behavioral Therapy in Schools* fills this gap both as a guide for training new practitioners in schools, and as a handbook of practical methods when applying strategies previously mastered. Covering a range of considerations including rationale for CBT, implementation, technology, and termination, *Applied Cognitive Behavioral Therapy in Schools* deserves a spot on every practitioner's bookshelf, if not on their desktop."

—**Eric Rossen**, PhD, NCSP, Director,
Professional Development & Standards,
National Association of School Psychologists

"New practitioners will love this book. As a trainer of school psychologists, I have seen new practitioners avoid providing therapy in the schools because they feel underprepared. Reading this book is like getting a CBT booster. It connects theory to practice within an MTSS framework while providing many examples, resources, and step-by-step guides for CBT implementation."

—**Heather Christian Martens**, PhD, Licensed Psychologist,
Associate Professor and Director of School Psychology Program,
Department of Psychology and Counseling, University of Central Arkansas

"*Applied Cognitive Behavioral Therapy in Schools* is a wonderful addition to the school psychology literature and is a must-have for early career school psychologists and students pursuing their graduate degrees. It brings a wealth of information and resources addressing research-based applications of CBT in school settings in a way that makes what is often seen as a complex and lengthy process doable and within reach for all."

—**Maria Wojtalewicz**, PhD, Child Psychologist,
Department of Defense Education Activity (DoDEA),
Stuttgart Region, Germany

"This book is a must-have resource for all mental health providers working in school settings. With chapters written by leading experts in the field of child psychology, this text provides school-based clinicians with the specific evidence-based strategies for supporting students presenting with a range of mental health symptoms and challenges."

—**Allison G. Dempsey**, PhD, Associate Professor; Director, Connections Program for High-Risk Infants and Families; Director of Informatics, Department of Psychiatry; Training Director, Post-Doctoral Fellowship Program in Clinical Health Psychology, Divisions of Adult Psychiatry and Child and Adolescent Mental Health, University of Colorado School of Medicine

"This book is a welcome treat for school mental health professionals. It provides state of the art ideas and application of CBT in an educational context. Chapters were succinctly written that strikes a balance of theory, research, and practice. The cases, discussion questions, worksheets, and handouts are invaluable resources for those who use CBT as therapeutic orientation in schools."

—**Carmelo Callueng**, PhD, Assistant Professor, School Psychology Program, Department of Educational Services and Leadership, Rowan University

"Drs. Joyce-Beaulieu and Zaboski set out to answer THE most pressing question about mental health problems in schools, i.e., "What can we do?" They have succeeded! In their well-researched and expertly edited book, *Applied Cognitive Behavioral Therapy in Schools*, they and the other expert contributors to this invaluable work have described demonstrably effective steps for ameliorating the mental health pandemic."

—**Ralph Eugene Cash**, PhD, ABPP, Professor, College of Psychology, Nova Southeastern University, Director, School-related Psychological Assessments and Clinical Interventions, (SPACI) Clinic, Past President of the National Association of School Psychologists

Applied Cognitive Behavioral Therapy in Schools

EDITED BY DIANA JOYCE-BEAULIEU

AND

BRIAN A. ZABOSKI

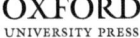

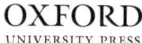

Oxford University Press is a department of the University of Oxford. It furthers
the University's objective of excellence in research, scholarship, and education
by publishing worldwide. Oxford is a registered trade mark of Oxford University
Press in the UK and certain other countries.

Published in the United States of America by Oxford University Press
198 Madison Avenue, New York, NY 10016, United States of America.

© Oxford University Press 2021

All rights reserved. No part of this publication may be reproduced, stored in
a retrieval system, or transmitted, in any form or by any means, without the
prior permission in writing of Oxford University Press, or as expressly permitted
by law, by license, or under terms agreed with the appropriate reproduction
rights organization. Inquiries concerning reproduction outside the scope of the
above should be sent to the Rights Department, Oxford University Press, at the
address above.

You must not circulate this work in any other form
and you must impose this same condition on any acquirer.

Library of Congress Cataloging-in-Publication Data
Names: Joyce-Beaulieu, Diana, editor. | A. Zaboski, Brian, editor.
Title: Applied cognitive behavioral therapy in schools /
edited by Diana Joyce-Beaulieu and Brian A. Zaboski.
Description: New York : Oxford University Press, [2021] |
Includes bibliographical references and index.
Identifiers: LCCN 2020056997 (print) | LCCN 2020056998 (ebook) |
ISBN 9780197581384 (paperback) | ISBN 9780197581407 (epub) | ISBN 9780197581414
Subjects: LCSH: Cognitive therapy for children. | Cognitive therapy for teenagers. |
School mental health services.
Classification: LCC RJ505.C63 A67 2021 (print) | LCC RJ505.C63 (ebook) |
DDC 618.92/891425—dc23
LC record available at https://lccn.loc.gov/2020056997
LC ebook record available at https://lccn.loc.gov/2020056998

DOI: 10.1093/med-psych/9780197581384.001.0001

This book is dedicated to Brooke, Lila, Aubrey, and Samantha Beaulieu and Caroline and Zachary Kenyon. They embrace every day in their young lives with cheerful anticipation. Their effervescent personalities are a welcomed reminder that life can be approached with wonderment and joy each day.

Diana Joyce-Beaulieu

For my daughter Jemma, who throughout this project learned to talk and began to walk and now runs—"fast!" Thank you for giving your daddy some of your time.

Brian A. Zaboski

CONTENTS

Foreword ix
Preface xiii
About the Editors xv
Contributors xvii

1. CBT Applications in Schools 1
   Diana Joyce-Beaulieu, Brian A. Zaboski, and Alexa R. Dixon

2. Theory and Research 25
   Brian A. Zaboski, Emma Romaker, and Diana Joyce-Beaulieu

3. Counseling Preparation 47
   Diana Joyce-Beaulieu and Brian A. Zaboski

4. Culturally Responsive Mental Health Services 65
   Janise S. Parker, Diana Joyce-Beaulieu, and Brian A. Zaboski

5. Psychoeducation, Relaxation Training, and Mindfulness 83
   Anna Schrack, Emma Romaker, Diana Joyce-Beaulieu, and Brian A. Zaboski

6. Core CBT Components: Part I 101
   Lee N. Purvis, Brian A. Zaboski, and Diana Joyce-Beaulieu

7. Core CBT Components: Part II 117
   Erin K. Reid, Leslie K. Taylor, Kelly N. Banneyer, Jose Dominguez, Gary Liu, Laurel L. Williams, Brian A. Zaboski, Sophie C. Schneider, and Eric A. Storch

8. Integrating Technology into School-Based Interventions 143
   Greg M. Muller, Brian A. Zaboski, and Diana Joyce-Beaulieu

9. Terminating Therapy and Referrals 163
   Jason Gallant, Diana Joyce-Beaulieu, and Brian A. Zaboski

Appendix: Quick Resources, Worksheets, and Handouts 181
Index 201

FOREWORD

The training of mental health practitioners, particularly those who will work with school-aged youth, is a complex and often arduous process. This training does not end (or begin) with formal graduate schooling but represents a lifelong commitment to learning and growth. Selecting instructional resources to support and inform such a journey can be a daunting task—for instructors, students, supervisors, and practitioners. Although describing an "ideal" text is difficult, the educational literature is rife with examples that fall woefully short of the mark.

An illuminating experiment might include a series of visits—to practicing clinicians, school-based supervisors, veteran instructors and professors, and perhaps graduate student study rooms—to peruse their bookshelves. We aren't interested in the glossy and shallow promotional materials that likely have never been opened, nor are we seeking the stuffy and arcane tomes that were procured to demonstrate credibility or professional status (and likely are covered in dust).

No, we are looking for the well-worn, bookmarked, and highlighted (often coffee-stained) works that never seem to make their way back to the shelf. You will find them propped open on a desk for reference, wedged in a backpack or computer bag, or on loan to students or colleagues. These are the one or two books that someone recommended to you, that you repeatedly purchase additional copies of (because you never seem to get them back when you loan them out), whose titles you easily remember due to the frequency with which you recommend them to others. What you are holding in your hands will rapidly find its way into your bag (or someone else's when you loan it out).

Applied Cognitive Behavioral Therapy in Schools excels in terms of depth of content, although this is not what sets it apart from other texts. Similarly, the laser focus on evidence-based applications of CBT within educational settings is a welcome change from broader, less applied treatments of school-based mental health. However, the "magic ingredient" as it were is the approach taken by the editors and chapter authors in providing information that is useful throughout the entirety of the training journey.

As might be expected given the graduate teaching experience of several contributors, *Applied Cognitive Behavioral Therapy in Schools* supports the foundational training of students with respect to effective mental health assessment, evaluation, and treatment—areas often given brief and shallow coverage in school psychology, counseling, and social work preparation programs. However, the text also offers critical thoughts on the culture and climate of educational/school settings, an area sorely neglected within the clinical and counseling psychology training pipelines. As such, a strong theoretical basis from which to conceptualize mental health and wellness is offered, and there is a rich discussion as to what constitutes a psychiatric or psychological disorder (and how to effectively differentiate psychopathology from developmental delays or abnormalities). Most impressive in this area is the vibrant backdrop that consistently relates the content back to the multiple roles and missions of public education and schools.

In the transition from graduate coursework to the variety of settings in which we practice—many school-based, even more outside of the traditional building—burgeoning practitioners face a number of barriers related to bringing theoretical knowledge into applied situations. *Applied Cognitive Behavioral Therapy in Schools* provides a wealth of material critical to university- and school-based internship supervision. Beyond the coverage we would expect related to ethical considerations and questions of client identification, there are numerous case-based examples of symptom presentation, functional impairment, setting events, cognitive distortions, emotional dysregulation, and disruptive behaviors. Perhaps more unusual and useful are the applied examples—many case-based, others more general—of treatment materials, including psychoeducational information, hierarchy-building techniques, exposure/avoidance activities, and behavior activation tasks.

From the standpoint of early career professionals—and those responsible for their continuing education—readers of *Applied Cognitive Behavioral Therapy in Schools* will find a consistently in-depth and realistic discussion of the real-world function that schools serve in childhood development, as well as clarification of the duty our mental health providers have with respect to student education. From an administrative stance, the text is unique in providing a thorough and easy-to-understand introduction to the tension and balance between decreasing resources and increasing needs, which undergird decision-making and resource allocation matrices such as Response to Intervention and Multi-Tiered Systems of Support. These materials are invaluable in understanding educational expectations, establishing effective goals, and evaluating performance within the educational environment.

A common question and concern among providers in almost any setting (but particularly for school-based clinicians) is how to find materials appropriate for providing relevant and accurate information to students, parents/families, teachers, or support staff. This issue has become increasingly important in a world where inaccurate or misleading information is easy to access and proliferate. Practitioners will find within *Applied Cognitive Behavioral Therapy in Schools* a variety of normalization/externalization materials appropriate for students (from elementary school to adult education), materials providing warning signs and suggestions or tips for parents and families, and various evidence-based classroom management techniques for their instructional colleagues that are easily applied at the whole-class (Tier 1), small-group (Tier 2), and individual (Tier 3) level as needed.

It is beyond rare to find a source of information and materials that has been designed and written specifically for school-based mental health training and preparation programs. The editors and chapter contributors of *Applied Cognitive Behavioral Therapy in Schools* are well-known experts in their respective fields, their discussions are clear and informative, and they have provided a wealth of cogent, evidence-based examples that lifelong learners will find critical to success throughout their journey. Drs. Joyce-Beaulieu and Zaboski have compiled the definitive example of a text we will find—well-worn, dog-eared, and coffee-stained—on bookshelves, in bags, and on desks for many years to come.

Joshua Nadeau, PhD
Clinical Director, Rogers Behavioral Health—Tampa

PREFACE

A little over a century ago there were no school psychologists in the United States. And only a generation past did school psychology see the development of the National Association of School Psychologists in 1969. With a quarter of students experiencing mental health needs during their education, mental health problems often arising during school-aged years, and most students unable or unwilling to seek help, many practitioners—novice and veteran alike—are left asking, What we can we do? The primary goal of the text is to describe an effective, efficient, and evidence-based answer to this question: cognitive behavioral therapy (CBT).

In Chapter 1 we present the sobering prevalence rates of mental health problems among school-aged youth and emphasize that mental health problems often endure into adulthood. We discuss the current infrastructure for addressing these concerns, including multilevel supports in schools, and explain how counseling is embedded within it.

In Chapter 2, we introduce CBT within a historical backdrop of famous thinkers with their own solutions to mental health problems. We argue that CBT is the most robust of these competing theoretical orientations, unpack its theoretical development, and provide an overview of CBT's research support and applications for children and adolescents.

Chapter 3 prepares readers to implement CBT by highlighting ethical and legal matters that arise in school-based counseling. We describe the professional ethics codes that guide practitioners as they deliver interventions in schools. The chapter also compares the benefits and drawbacks of group versus individual therapy and introduces the micro skills essential to effective service delivery.

Culturally responsive therapy receives a thorough treatment in Chapter 4, which offers strategies for incorporating racial, ethnic, and developmental client characteristics into CBT intervention plans. Readers will learn how to acknowledge these characteristics as important and personal sources of client strength that can improve therapeutic alliances and intervention outcomes.

Chapter 5 establishes some of the more general elements of CBT: psychoeducation, relaxation training, problem solving, motivational interviewing, and mindfulness.

Here practitioners will learn some easily implemented counseling techniques that can be flexibly applied to referral problems within a CBT framework.

Chapters 6 and 7 contain CBT's core intervention techniques—what many researchers and practitioners consider CBT's active treatment ingredients. Chapter 6 explores behavioral activation and cognitive restructuring, two essential skills for managing a plethora of concerns, including depression and anxiety. Chapter 7 focuses on CBT for anxiety and trauma, specifically attending to exposure and response prevention and its application in school settings.

Mobile devices, apps, iPads, and virtual reality are just a handful of the technological advancements in the 21st century. Chapter 8 provides a technological perspective on CBT, presenting ideas and advice for practitioners looking to integrate technology into practice. Chapter 8 also offers advice to help practitioners navigate the mobile mental health apps on the market.

Chapter 9 addresses closure, a necessary but often overlooked element of counseling. Here we discuss how best to conclude CBT and conduct booster sessions. As a practical matter, we also acknowledge that school-based CBT may not always meet a client's needs. To this end, we recommend multidisciplinary consultation options and a continuum of referral options ranging from outpatient settings to residential treatment facilities. Lastly, the Appendix offers quick resources including counseling worksheets, parent handouts, and an extensive listing of therapy apps.

School-based services have evolved considerably over the last century thanks to the intrepid practitioners and researchers who voiced the novel—and perhaps societally dubious—idea that children and adolescents need help, too. Through numerous resources, careful research, and unique case examples, we hope that this practical text will guide a new cohort of practitioners to discover the rewards and challenges of school-based mental health.

ABOUT THE EDITORS

Diana Joyce-Beaulieu is a Scholar at the National Association of School Psychologist-approved and American Psychological Association-accredited School Psychology Program at the University of Florida (UF). She has taught numerous graduate courses including developmental psychopathology, social-emotional assessment, and cognitive behavioral therapy. As a licensed Psychologist and nationally certified School Psychologist, she administers the practica program and supervises graduate students with placements across five county school districts and five clinical sites. Clinical sites have included a child morbid obesity clinic, an adolescence diabetes treatment compliance clinic, a hospital psychiatric unit, a juvenile residential treatment facility, a behavioral health center, a disability center for college students, and UF's PK Yonge Developmental Research School. Her research interests include behavioral/conduct disorders and intensive mental health intervention. Her publications include five books, 30 chapters, and numerous peer-reviewed articles. She has served as co-principal investigator for state and national training grants focused on mental health supports within a Multi-tiered Systems of Support (MTSS) model.

Brian A. Zaboski is a licensed Connecticut psychologist and a Nationally Certified School Psychologist. He completed his PhD in School Psychology at the University of Florida, where he gained clinical experience with children and adults across a continuum of care ranging from school-based to acute inpatient facilities. He has considerable expertise in cognitive behavioral therapy (CBT) for a panoply of psychological disorders, and proficiency in educational, psychological, and neuropsychological assessment. He developed a clinical and research specialty in CBT with exposure at Rogers Behavioral Health under the supervision of Eric Storch, as well as during his clinical postdoctoral studies in the University of Florida's Department of Psychiatry, Division of Psychology. As the Associate Director for Clinical Psychology at the Yale OCD Research Clinic, his primary interests include the application of sophisticated quantitative methods to understanding the neurobiological networks of individuals afflicted with OCD, improving exposure therapy through translational neuroscience, and training clinicians in exposure-based techniques.

CONTRIBUTORS

Kelly N. Banneyer, PhD
Department of Pediatrics
Baylor College of Medicine
Houston, TX, USA

Alexa R. Dixon, MEd
School of Special Education, School Psychology and Early Childhood Studies
University of Florida
Gainesville, FL, USA

Jose Dominguez, MPH
Menninger Department of Psychiatry and Behavioral Sciences
Baylor College of Medicine
Houston, TX, USA

Jason Gallant, PhD
Boys Town Central Florida Behavioral Health Clinic
Orlando, FL, USA

Gary Liu, PhD
Menninger Department of Psychiatry and Behavioral Sciences
Baylor College of Medicine
Houston, TX, USA

Greg M. Muller, PhD
University of Florida, Health Psychology—Springhill
Gainesville, FL, USA

Janise S. Parker, PhD
School Psychology and Counselor Education
College of William & Mary
Williamsburg, VA, USA

Lee N. Purvis, PhD
Department of Psychology
Louisiana State University
Shreveport, LA, USA

Erin K. Reid, MEd
Department of Psychological, Health, and Learning Sciences
University of Houston
Houston, TX, USA

Emma Romaker, BA
Department of Psychiatry
Yale University
New Haven, CT, USA

Sophie C. Schneider, PhD
Menninger Department of Psychiatry and Behavioral Sciences
Baylor College of Medicine
Houston, TX, USA

Anna Schrack, PhD
Rice Psychology Group
Tampa, FL, USA

Eric A. Storch, PhD
Menninger Department of Psychiatry
   and Behavioral Sciences
Baylor College of Medicine
Houston, TX, USA

Leslie K. Taylor, PhD
Department of Psychiatry
University of Texas Health Sciences
   Center at Houston
Houston, TX, USA

Laurel L. Williams, DO
Menninger Department of Psychiatry
   and Behavioral Sciences
Baylor College of Medicine
Houston, TX, USA

1

CBT Applications in Schools

DIANA JOYCE-BEAULIEU, BRIAN A. ZABOSKI, AND
ALEXA R. DIXON ■

Within the United States, it is estimated that 20% of school-aged children will experience significant mental health needs at some time during their education (Kessler et al., 2005; Merikangas et al., 2010; U.S. Department of Health and Human Services [USDHHS], 2000). Among students ages 9 to 17, approximately 21% will exhibit symptoms of a diagnosable disorder during the year, 11% will have significant impairment due to symptoms, and 5% will exhibit extreme functional impairment. For students (ages 10–24) served in schools across all disabilities, nearly 50% are mental health related (Gore et al., 2011). In a review of epidemiology studies published between 1993 and 2005, Costello et al. (2005) rank ordered median estimates for the most common mental health disorders among 5- to 17-year-olds. They found the highest prevalence for anxiety-related disorders (8%), followed by disruptive behavioral disorders (7%), major depression (4.8%), substance use (4.75%), conduct disorder (3.8%), oppositional defiant disorder (3.5%), attention-deficit/hyperactivity disorder (ADHD; 3%), simple phobias (2.5%), social phobia (2%), and separation anxiety (1.8%). Researchers examining other samples have also found high prevalence rates for learning disorders (9.7%), ADHD (9.5%), and stuttering (6.1%; Karpiak & Zaboski, 2013).

Another study reviewed 15 years of adolescent prevalence data and found that the prevalence of separation anxiety and ADHD decreases from childhood to adolescence, whereas the prevalence of depression and substance use disorders increases (Costello et al., 2011). In reviewing 30 years of longitudinal data for rural Appalachian students (primarily American Indian and Anglo), researchers concluded that most mental health disorders manifest in childhood and can precipitate adverse outcomes through adulthood (Costello et al., 2016). They also noted that 6 out of 10 (60%) children with early psychiatric disorders had adverse adult outcomes, including multiple mental health problems, suicidality, life-threatening health concerns, incarceration or felony charges, being fired from multiple jobs, lack of family/peer support, and high school dropout. In contrast, only 1 out of 5 (20%) individuals without childhood mental health diagnoses experienced adverse adult outcomes. The correlates and predictors of adult psychiatric and substance use disorders included family/environment risks, trauma, genetic markers, epigenetics, and poverty (irrespective of race/ethnicity). Together these studies provide a snapshot of the mental health needs school personnel are likely to serve, and these findings argue for early intervention supports.

Unmet mental health needs can have a significant negative impact on students' education and life opportunities. Nearly 44% will drop out before completing high school, and this statistic goes up to 50% for minority students (Greene & Winters, 2005). For secondary students, 46% of school failures are considered attributable to psychiatric disorders (Stoep et al., 2003). In considering the more serious consequences of acute mental health needs, suicide is the third leading cause of death for students ages 10 to 24 (Center for Disease and Prevention [CDCP], 2017). Overall, 16% of high schoolers have seriously considered suicide, 13% have made a plan, and 8% reported an attempt. Among youth completing suicide, 81% are males (CDCP, 2017). Given these outcomes, there is a need for early, high-quality mental health services for vulnerable youth.

Only 20% of children with diagnosable disorders receive mental health services, only 40% of those with serious emotional disorders receive care from a specialty mental health professional, and less than 10% receive treatment for more than 3 months (Costello et al., 2016). Most youth receiving services (70–80%) acquire intervention through their school district rather than clinics or private practitioners (American Academy of Pediatrics, 2004; Burns et al., 1995; Hoagwood & Erwin, 1997; Rones & Hoagman, 2000). Based on these findings, several national initiatives have advanced the role of schools in mental health service delivery for youth (President's New Freedom Commission on Mental Health, 2003). Some of the benefits of school-based counseling interventions include a reduced risk of counseling no-shows, elimination of insurance treatment limitations, and fewer transportation barriers for families. Schools also provide a naturalistic setting for counseling with abundant opportunities for in vivo practice and generalization of new skills, offer sustainable resources located within schools, and facilitate opportunities to increase parent involvement (Atkins et al., 2010).

EFFICACY OF COGNITIVE BEHAVIORAL THERAPY (CBT) IN SCHOOLS

In considering best practices and evidence-based counseling treatments, the Task Force on Promotion and Dissemination of Psychological Procedures through the American Psychological Association has designated CBT as "well established" for use in children and adolescents (Silverman et al., 2008). CBT has been applied with success in school settings to address the most common childhood/adolescent mental health syndromes, including anxiety-related disorders, phobias, depression, obsessive-compulsive disorder, ADHD, and behavioral/conduct disorders

(Ginsburg et al., 2008; Masia Warner et al., 2005, 2007; Mychailyszyn et al., 2011; Neil & Christensen, 2009; Parker et al., 2016).

For students with mental health needs, which may not include a formal diagnosis, there also are a range of validated counseling approaches, including psychoeducation, mindfulness, and scripted or modular cognitive behavioral curricula (Friedberg et al., 2009; Ginsburg et al., 2008; Masia Warner et al., 2005, 2007; Mychailyszyn et al., 2011; Neil & Christensen, 2009). A meta-analysis by Cuijpers et al. (2014) indicates that medication and counseling each independently exert moderate effects on improvement compared to placebo ($g = 0.35$, $g = 0.37$, respectively), suggesting that counseling can be an effective, viable, and side effect–free option compared to pharmacotherapy. Research also shows that CBT may have more long-term enduring results than medication alone (Canton et al., 2012; Carpenter et al., 2018; Cuijpers et al., 2013). Based on a review of 106 meta-analyses, some of the strongest CBT effects are for bulimia, anxiety and anger-related disorders (Hofmann et al., 2012), with even stronger effects when combined with exposure and response prevention (E/RP—discussed further in Chapter 7). When symptoms and impairment are acute or severe, studies indicate that medication outperforms counseling in the short term (Blanco et al., 2013; de Gage et al., 2012). However, augmenting medication with CBT increases intervention effects beyond medication alone ($g = 0.43$; Cuijpers et al., 2014). In addition to improving mental health status, school-based CBT has also resulted in secondary benefits including improved attendance, lower discipline referrals, and higher overall grade point average (GPA) (Michael et al., 2013). For these reasons, CBT remains an essential intervention choice for school-based practitioners (Zaboski et al., 2017).

As noted in this section, the level of mental health needs can be conceptualized in three categories: mild, moderate, and severe. It is also common in medicine to conceptualize patient care in a three-level paradigm: prevention, treatment, and rehabilitation (World Health Organization, 2001). In this medical framework, preventive actions interrupt the causes of illness, treatment recognizes emerging illness and stops symptoms from worsening, and rehabilitation tries to restore function to the greatest extent possible. Similar tiered models also have been developed for school systems' intervention design.

MULTI-TIERED SYSTEMS OF SUPPORT (MTSS)

MTSS is a comprehensive framework for providing levels of support for students based on their progress monitoring data and response to intervention (National Association of Directors of Special Education [NADSE], 2008a, 2008b). The MTSS framework is often conceptualized as a three-tier model, although variations exist (Figure 1.1). These tiers are based on students' assessed needs, and progress monitoring assessments are utilized across all tiers to evaluate student success. The model was created to address academic achievement, and its application has resulted in considerable improvement in core skills (Grapin et al,

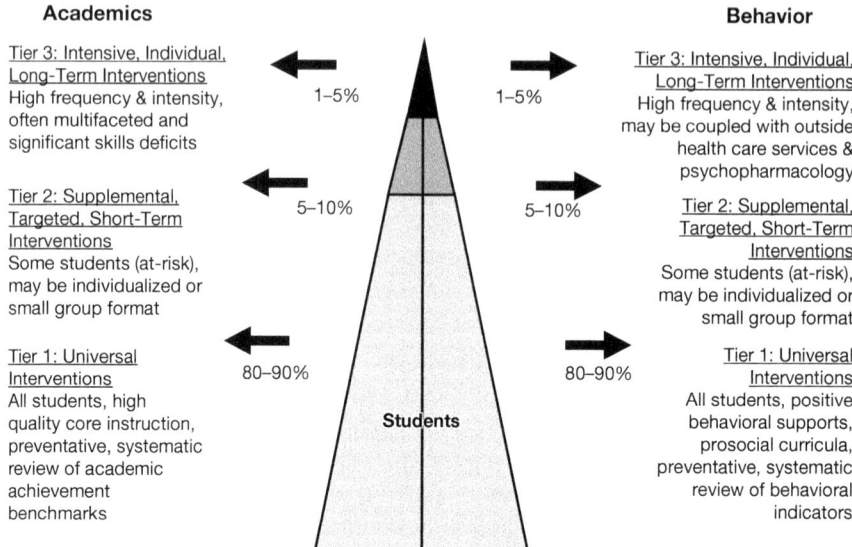

Figure 1.1 Three-Tiered Model of School Mental Health Supports (Adapted from Sprague, 2007)

2019). This framework also has been applied to behavioral and social-emotional functioning (NADSE, 2008a, 2008b; Sulkowski et al., 2011).

Tier 1

Tier 1 focuses on all students. Supports at this level are universal and include evidence-based, high-quality classroom instruction, social-emotional learning curricula, and classroom-wide behavioral management practices. Ideally, the needs of approximately 80% to 90% of students across behavioral, social-emotional, and academic domains should be met by these universally available supports. Like the tiered medical model, this tier is preventive. Group data are reviewed three or four times a year to ensure that most students are meeting benchmarks (e.g., grade-level vocabulary acquisition, math skills, absences under the state mean, no discipline referrals or suspensions). When less than 80% of students are achieving expectations, it suggests that the curricula or the system's infrastructure may need adjustment. The exercise of reviewing broad group data may also reveal patterns of need for specific groups (e.g., minority or homeless children) that the school infrastructure needs to address at Tier 1 (Sulkowski & Joyce-Beaulieu, 2014). If group patterns exist, it also may be unfair to isolate those children for Tier 2 or 3 services when there are systemic-level changes that could ameliorate difficulties (e.g., more culturally appropriate curricula for diverse students, bus pickup at homeless shelters, quick implementation of free lunch for temporary circumstances such as homelessness). Another approach to acquiring group social-emotional data is the use of universal screeners (Joyce-Beaulieu &

Zaboski, in press). These instruments are typically brief rating scales and identify students at risk. Forms are often completed by teachers.

As an example, if greater than 20% of children are not meeting basic reading skills, perhaps a better curriculum, more instruction time, or different instructional methods are needed. Likewise, if 20% of students are receiving behavioral referrals or exhibiting high absenteeism, it suggests that classroom management strategies and attendance policies need review. Diligent review of a school's whole-group data ensures accountability for maintaining high-quality pedagogy that is responsive to the needs of the population the school is serving (Benner et al., 2013). Monitoring the school's ability to meet students' needs while simultaneously identifying those students who require early intervention offers the additional benefit of closing the disparity in services for minority students (Benner et al., 2013). When the needs of 80% or more of the students are met, those whose scores remain low are provided Tier 2 interventions to quickly close the achievement or behavioral functioning gap (Fixsen et al., 2005).

Tier 2

The second tier provides supplemental, targeted interventions and supports for at-risk students. These interventions are short term and highly efficient and are considered a rapid response to emerging risk. Often a small-group format is utilized for children with common needs. For example, in elementary schools there are often clusters of students who could benefit from social skills development, test anxiety reduction, or self-regulation techniques. At Tier 2, CBT may be applied using treatment protocols or scripted or modular curricula. Counseling groups may address these needs, sometimes in tandem with classroom behavior incentive plans. Progress monitoring data are collected during small-group interventions and used to make decisions regarding whether interventions have been successful, need to be continued, or need to be changed. Assessments may include several options, such as observational data, naturally occurring school data (e.g., grades, attendance, frequency of nurse visits, behavioral referrals, suspensions), rating scales, and Subjective Units of Distress Scale (SUDS) measurement. Intervention frequency (how many sessions per week), intensity (length of sessions), and duration (total number of weeks) can all be adjusted. If a student's progress is not adequate, additional interventions may be added, including progression to the Tier 3 level.

Tier 3

Tier 3 interventions are intensive, often multifaceted, and typically delivered individually (Eagle et al., 2014). Some Tier 3 interventions, however, may be delivered in groups, especially when the student's symptoms or impairment, like social anxiety, could be remediated from social interaction (Zaboski et al., 2019). For mental health and social-emotional needs, Tier 3 may involve more formalized CBT techniques and sessions that are highly customized to the student (e.g., modified CBT for autism; Zaboski & Storch, 2018). Collaboration with outside care providers and pharmacological treatment may also be indicated depending on symptom severity (Wexler, 2017). Tier 3 interventions also require progress monitoring, so the use of pathology rating scales (e.g., anxiety, depression, conduct disorder, oppositional defiant disorder, and obsessive-compulsive disorder) in additional to school performance improvement measures (e.g., attendance, behavioral discipline referrals) is common.

Despite being provided high-quality core instruction and social-emotional supports as well as significant Tier 2 and 3 interventions, a small percentage of students will need additional supports on a sustained, long-term basis. For these students, schools may initiate eligibility for special education procedures and consideration for placement as emotional disturbance (ED), as well as refer them to providers outside of the school system for additional supports.

SECTION 504 PLANS, INDIVIDUALS WITH DISABILITIES EDUCATION ACT (IDEA), AND INDIVIDUALIZED EDUCATION PROGRAMS (IEPS)

Section 504 Plans

Section 504 plans offer protections for individuals with disabilities and originated with the Rehabilitation Act of 1973 (1973). The broad legislation is a civil rights law passed by Congress and applies to individuals of all ages in a range of settings, including employment and schools. The Americans with Disabilities Act of 1990 (1990) and the Americans with Disabilities Act Amendment Act of 2008 (ADAAA, 2008) were subsequently passed to update the law's provisions. These laws offer additional guidance on Section 504 plans as they apply to educational settings. The core principle ensures an equal opportunity for individuals with disabilities to access programs, activities, and advancement. For schools, this includes participation in all school-based activities (e.g., access to quality instruction/learning, including extracurricular activities such as sports or drama). Eligibility criteria require that:

1. The student has a physical or mental impairment that interferes with one or more daily life activities,
2. The student has a record of this impairment, or
3. The student is regarded as having the impairment.

School decisions on whether a student meets Section 504 criteria may be based on a range of information sources. Eligibility teams may review education data, attendance, discipline referrals, test score history, and documentation of diagnoses from healthcare providers and also may supplement this information with assessments to gather more information. However, qualifying for a 504 plan does not require a formalized assessment battery the way that qualifying for special education would. This is an important point, as it is one area of differentiation from the criteria for special education placement.

The Section 504 definition of a physical impairment includes those that are the result of a physical disorder or condition, cosmetic disfigurement, or anatomical loss that impact a physiological system, such as musculoskeletal, digestive, or neurological. Mental impairment is included and can be a diagnosed mental illness, emotional impairment, or a specific learning disability. Major life activities include care of oneself, breathing, speaking, or working. In the classroom, this can also include concentrating, thinking, or communicating (U.S. Department of Education, Office of Civil Rights, n.d.). Section 504 plans are written with school personnel and parental input and include accommodations and modifications to ensure students can access the curricula and school activities. At times, these plans may request supplemental counseling support services within the school. These plans are reviewed periodically but do not have measurable goals as would be required for special education placement plans.

IDEA and IEPs

Provisions through the IDEA and the IDEA Improvement Act of 2004 include 14 categories for special education services (IDEA, 1990, 2004): autism, deaf-blindness, deafness, developmental delay, ED, hearing impairment, intellectual disability, multiple disabilities, orthopedic impairment, other health impairment (OHI), specific learning disability, speech or language impairment, traumatic brain injury, and visual impairment including blindness. Across the United States approximately 7.1 million children receive special education services, which represents 14% of all students (National Center for Education Statistics, 2020).

Special education placement requires an eligibility assessment and development of an IEP, a plan that incorporates supportive accommodations and modifications tailored to the student's needs (Office of Special Education and Rehabilitative Services, U.S. Department of Education, 2000). Goals and outcome measures are written into the plans and progress is monitored by the school's problem-solving team so plans can be adapted as needed. The IEP differs from a Section 504 plan in that formalized annual review meetings are required (more often if parents request them) and reevaluation is required every 3 years. If the student's disability is short term, the school-based eligibility team also may withdraw the special education designation once all goals are met. If the needs are related to social-emotional struggles, behavioral disorders, chronic health syndromes, or mental health diagnoses, designated services often include counseling. For students with mental health support needs, specific counseling goals, progress monitoring mechanisms, and frequency, intensity, and duration qualifiers may also be included. As noted in Chapter 3, these specified IEP requirements will need to be followed and documented when planning counseling sessions. Additionally, students in any IDEA category, even if it is not primarily mental health related, may have counseling as a supplemental support depending on their needs. As an example, a child who has suffered a sudden loss of vision may need long-term special education services under the category of visual impairment. This child also may need shorter-term counseling for emotional supports associated with depression and adjusting to this new life circumstance.

The IDEA categories that might be most amenable for counseling include ED and OHI when related to the stress of chronic health conditions. It is important to note that these categories do not necessarily align well with mental health diagnoses from the *Diagnostic and Statistical Manual of Mental Disorders* (DSM; American Psychiatric Association, 2013), although many diagnoses can be served within the broad IDEA designations. This may be a point of confusion for parents and outside service providers less familiar with school-based services, especially when a diagnosis is documented and needs are obvious. Part of the role of school personnel, making eligibility decisions, is to understand the overlap between DSM and educational taxonomies and ensure students are placed appropriately.

ED

When significant social-emotional needs manifest, the ED category may be designated. Within special education, 5% of students have this designation (National Center for Education Statistics, 2020). The criteria for ED are defined in IDEA (2004, Sec. 300.8 (c) (4)):

> Emotional Disturbance means a condition exhibiting one or more of the following characteristics over a long period of time and to a marked degree that adversely affects a child's educational performance:
> (A) An inability to learn that cannot be explained by intellectual, sensory, or health factors.
> (B) An inability to build or maintain satisfactory interpersonal relationships with peers and teachers.
> (C) Inappropriate types of behavior or feelings under normal circumstances.
> (D) A general pervasive mood of unhappiness or depression.
> (E) A tendency to develop physical symptoms or fears associated with personal or school problems.

Eligibility requires a formal assessment establishing the criteria and a team decision. Students with ED are a heterogeneous group. Thus, the term may be viewed as an umbrella label encompassing a range of externalizing and internalizing difficulties. Externalizers often include conduct dysregulation difficulties (e.g., intermittent explosive disorder, oppositional defiant disorder, conduct disorders). Internalizers may include anxiety-related or mood disorders (e.g., phobias, social anxiety, generalized anxiety, bipolar disorder, depression). Depending on the severity, children with other syndromes may also receive special education services under ED (e.g., obsessive-compulsive disorder, eating disorders, schizophrenia).

It is important to note that although some DSM diagnoses are mentioned as examples in this text, having the diagnosis does not automatically qualify students for services; they would still need to meet criteria A to E as noted by IDEA (2004). Likewise, students may exhibit significant emotional disturbance without meeting criteria for a DSM diagnosis and still be eligible for special education ED services. As noted previously, this can be confusing to parents, especially if they have been referred by a private provider with a recommendation for special education and a documented diagnosis. If the mental health syndrome does not have the impairments noted in the criteria, the child may not qualify for special education. Individual states also have additional special education statutes and procedures to consider. Given the nature of ED, it is likely that IEPs will require counseling to address at least some portion of the youth's functioning.

OHI

The designation of OHI is often utilized for students with chronic health illnesses. Examples include ADHD, heart conditions, tuberculosis, rheumatic fever, nephritis, asthma, sickle cell anemia, hemophilia, epilepsy, lead poisoning, leukemia, diabetes, or any other medical condition, such as Tourette syndrome (IDEA, 2004). The OHI criteria include limited strength, vitality, or alertness, including a heightened alertness with respect to the educational environment due to chronic or acute health problems that adversely affects a student's educational performance. A medical assessment documenting the health problem is required (IDEA, 2004). OHI accounts for about 15% of all children receiving special education services (National Center for Education Statistics, 2020). For students receiving OHI services, counseling would most likely be supplemental rather than the primary intervention and would be related to the stressors and coping mechanisms for illness.

Chronic Health Conditions

Approximately 20% of youth are diagnosed with a chronic illness (e.g., diabetes, asthma, epilepsy), and of those children, 6.5% have illnesses that significantly interfere with normal school activities (Merikangas et al., 2015, 2010; USDHHS, 2007). More severe forms of illnesses may be related to discrete medical interventions (e.g., corrective spinal surgeries) or ongoing treatment (e.g., multiple rounds of chemotherapy for leukemia with episodes of remission and relapse, cardiovascular disorders). Chronic illness is defined as lasting at least 3 months, requiring extensive medical care, and negatively impacting the ability to participate in typical activities (Mokkink et al., 2008). For these students, Section 504 plans or IEPs under the special education category of OHI provisions may be implemented. However, a nationwide survey found that 504 plans are most often utilized for individuals with ADHD, chronic health conditions, and multiple diagnoses and impairments (Holler & Zirkel, 2008). Accommodations and modifications for students with chronic health struggles often include significant allowances for medical absences, additional time for making up class assignments or credits, streamlining curricula, additional breaks for fatigue, and counseling, and in more serious circumstances, a hospital-homebound provision may include sending a teacher to the child's home for instruction. Adding to the complexity of service needs for these students, research has indicated that 70% of students with special medical needs have three or more comorbid conditions (Parasuraman et al., 2018).

Studies of youth with chronic health conditions indicate that they have a higher incidence of some behavioral, academic, cognitive, and social-emotional difficulties (Clark et al., 1999; Maslow et al., 2011; Reuben & Pastor, 2013; Shaw & McGabe, 2008; Shiu, 2001). Research has also suggested a link between poor physical health and a variety of mental health needs (Merikangas et al., 2015, 2010; USDHHS, 2007). But the area of impact may differ by the illness and the severity of impairment. In a meta-analysis, Boekaerts and Roder (1999) reviewed 200 studies and found that children with chronic illness exhibited more behavioral problems associated with depression and social withdrawal. A meta-analysis of 569 studies in 2010 (Pinquart & Shen, 2011) noted higher externalizing ($g = 0.22$), internalizing ($g = 0.47$), and total behavioral problems ($g = 0.42$) on the Child Behavioral Checklist (CBCL; Achenbach & Rescorla, 2001) for students with chronic illness as compared to students without chronic illness. Total effects were moderate for the teacher-report forms ($g = 0.37$) and small ($g = 0.17$) for the child self-report forms of the CBCL. Interestingly, the highest internalizing scores were for children with chronic fatigue syndrome ($g = 1.42$), while some of the highest externalizing scores were for students with epilepsy ($g = 0.88$ to $g = 1.07$). A national longitudinal survey of 22,831 children in Canada found those with chronic illness were more likely to have high absenteeism, learning disabilities, and mental health conditions (McDougall et al., 2004). Effects were most impairing for children with chronic illnesses that limited physical activity. A review of another large sample of students in California ($N = 22,730$, 2nd to 11th grades) found that chronic health problems increased the probability of low performance on a standardized English test by 55% and math scores by 56% (Crump et al., 2013).

When planning counseling for students with chronic illness, there are several unique considerations. For students without illness, counseling content is usually provided sequentially with a set schedule. However, for children with high absences due to medical procedures and who have fatigue, pain management, or reduced concentration factors, counseling will need to be highly flexible. Gaps in attendance may require reestablishing rapport, reviewing prior concepts and strategies, and taking frequent breaks during sessions. Counseling also may need to prioritize general encouragement and a nurturing stance for the child. Lastly, when notified that a child's condition is terminal, the school and parents will likely advise changing the counseling focus to a palliative care model. This involves acknowledging the strengths the child has, facilitating their choices in how they will spend their remaining time with school friends and family, and supporting their psychological and social needs. Schools will withdraw counseling goals related to academic achievement, making up missed work, or preparing for high-stakes testing and follow the child and parents' lead on when and if child wishes to continue attending school.

In summary, this chapter has provided an overview of the national prevalence trends for youth with mental health needs and supporting evidence for delivery of CBT in schools. The MTSS model and the ways in which tiered services are integrated within the context of school referral processes were reviewed. For more intensive needs, Section 504 and IDEA provisions also may offer formalized accommodation and modification supports that include counseling intervention. The students most likely to acquire longer-term services include those with ED, OHI, and chronic health conditions. Together, this information offers a context for school-based CBT.

SAMPLE SCHOOL-BASED COUNSELING REPORT

The counseling case report provided here offers an overview of how increasing intervention intensity over time might be provided within a school utilizing an MTSS model for mild to moderate level of need. Later chapters will provide embedded counseling examples for more intensive needs as specific techniques are introduced, and by the end of this text readers will learn how conceptualize and apply CBT in cases like these and monitor the progress of students.

Tier 2 Counseling Intervention Summary
This report contains privileged and confidential information and may only be released with written parental consent except as provided by law.

Child's Name: Kaveh (pseudonym)   Parents:
Date of Birth (DOB):   Date of Initial Contact: 2-7-2021
Chronological Age (CA): 11-2   Date of Final Contact: 3-30-2021
Counselor: Grade: 6th

Reason for Referral

Kaveh was referred for counseling following an Individual Education Program (IEP) meeting. His teachers and mother specifically expressed behavioral concerns in regards to having exceptionally high personal performance expectations, self-derogatory comments, becoming easily frustrated, and being unable to cope adequately.

Background Information

Kaveh is an 11-year-old who resides with his biological parents. English is the only language spoken in the home. He attended the same elementary school from kindergarten through 5th grade and transitioned to 6th-grade middle school this year. In kindergarten, the school speech therapist identified a speech impairment for which Kaveh received 60 minutes of speech therapy each week. In 1st grade, Kaveh also qualified for gifted services and subsequently began receiving enrichment classes. He has maintained grades of A's and B's since kindergarten.

The counselor's review of school records indicates Kaveh's kindergarten teacher noted he was a quick learner and high achiever but had difficulty controlling frustration, rapidly becoming angry if things did not go as he expected. As a result, parents, teachers, and the school counselor met during a problem-solving team meeting and discussed the following intervention strategies: allowing Kaveh time to "cool down," discussing and rehearsing ways to obtain desired items by raising his hand, offering alternative methods for expressing anger (e.g., asking teacher for help), and encouraging Kaveh to take a deep breathing break when upset. The counselor noted in his record that his behavior improved, with fewer outbursts. In 1st grade, Kaveh's parents initiated outside counseling services through a local family behavioral support clinic. He learned a three-step program (ALERT) to calm himself and manage his aggression: thinking calming thoughts, breathing ("blow out the bad thought"), and making good choices. In collaboration with parents, the classroom teachers reminded Kaveh to use ALERT as needed. There were only minor outbursts throughout the year. In the spring of 3rd grade, Kaveh's outbursts increased again and the problem-solving team, in collaboration with the speech/language therapist, added a weekly small-group social pragmatics intervention. Specifically, he was taught how to adaptively express his feelings and emotions and self-monitor his anger. Progress monitoring data in his record indicated that the intervention lowered outbursts to zero by the 9th week. In 4th grade, school team members reviewed Kaveh's IEP and concluded that he had met all speech goals, behaviorally matured, and progressed with his appropriate peer interactions. He no longer met criteria for speech impaired, so his IEP for speech services was closed, exiting him from special education. No behavioral incidents were noted for 5th grade.

Description and Analysis of the Problem

Teacher Interview

Kaveh transferred from elementary to middle school in 6th grade. His current teachers note he is a hardworking student with exceptional math skills who places considerable stress on himself to achieve and never get a wrong answer. They also noted he has found middle school curricula challenging in some classes, including science and language arts. His teachers are concerned that he becomes easily upset when he does not understand a new concept the first time it is presented or when asked how he would find an answer. Specifically, they noted a variety of triggers leading to his frustrations, including missing needed items (e.g., pencil, journal) or forgetting something (e.g., lunch money); situations that challenge him (e.g., group work when he is not always right and wants to compete), time constraints (e.g., tests), and believing he should have done better (e.g., assignment, test); and social situations where he feels annoyed by other students. The teachers also mentioned that when Kaveh becomes frustrated he typically reacts with negative self-talk (e.g., curses; "I'm stupid"; "I should be able to do this easy"; "I'm never gonna pass this").

At this time he has three behavioral referrals for directing his aggression to others when he becomes frustrated (e.g., verbal insults, physically pushing). Data indicate in the last 3 weeks he has had at least one outburst a day and one aggressive act every week. Teacher strategies have included asking him to take a time out for 3 minutes, discussing his behavior with him once he is calm, and ignoring his minor frustrations (e.g., mumbling, grimacing) if they are not interrupting other students. One teacher mentioned that most other students in the class react to Kaveh's behavior by staying away from him, and she is worried about peer neglect as he adjusts to this new cohort. Teachers also indicated that Kaveh can be reasoned with when not angry and very apologetic to others for his behaviors once he calms down.

Parent Interview

The counselor interviewed Kaveh's mother regarding her concerns about his behavior. She indicated that Kaveh has unrealistic expectations and that they are leading to his frustration and meltdowns. She shared that he becomes frustrated easily at home, like when he did not perform a new stunt on his skateboard correctly the first time or when he had to study more than usual to keep up with classwork. She added that when he has a bad day, he talks "nonsense" (e.g., that he will never get into a good college, never get a great job, and just be a loser in life). Despite these challenges, he has several strengths, like his love of family, soccer, skateboarding, and video games. He has several close friends in the neighborhood who enjoy these activities with him. His mother's goals are for him to more frequently ask for help, pause to get his composure before acting out, and think less self-critically.

Observations

During classroom observations, it was noted that Kaveh is on task about 80% of the time and polite to teachers. He also seems to have a few casual friends who he engages with between classes. His book bag and work folders are somewhat disheveled, making it difficult for him to locate things at times. When work is difficult his body tenses, he gently bangs his head on the desk or against the wall, or he puts his torso under the table to escape the situation. He also softly mutters some self-derogatory statements ("Can't get this stupid stuff"; "My dumb brain lost the pencil again"; "This is hopeless"). If peers tell him to "chill out" or "be quiet," he will sharply reply "shut up."

Student Interview

A semistructured interview was conducted with Kaveh. He indicated that he becomes upset when he does not meet his own expectations. He labeled himself as a "perfectionist." He said that he knows he overreacts and has expectations that are too high and that do not help. Kaveh said math comes easy to him but science and language arts frustrate him (especially grammar). When asked to describe how those subjects are frustrating, he mentioned that when he encounters a scientific theory or has to memorize grammar rules, he gets nervous, his mind shuts down, he thinks he will never get it, and he calls himself "stupid." He likes facts in science but not theories because they are a "waste of time." He does not understand why grammar rules are more important than his creative ideas. Kaveh thinks he is smarter than his peers and does not like to be corrected or redirected. As a result, other students annoy him in class (especially a couple of male students) when they continually interrupt him or do not listen when he tells them to stop talking. Kaveh noted he wants to be the best or not bother, and he is secretly afraid that he will disappoint his family and not get into a great college if he cannot get everything right in 6th grade.

Assessment Measures

Kaveh's emotional and behavioral functioning was assessed using the Behavior Assessment System for Children, Third Edition—Teacher Rating Scale (BASC-3 TRS; Reynolds & Kamphaus, 2015) and Parent Rating Scale (BASC-3 PRS). The BASC-3 is an omnibus behavior rating scale designed to assess a broad range of children and adolescent behaviors and emotions. Preintervention, Kaveh's mother and father rated Kaveh's depression in the at-risk range, whereas his teacher rated it in the clinically significant range. Similarly, his teacher rated his anxiety in the clinically significant range, and his parents rated it in the at-risk range. All other clinical scales on the BASC-3 were average range. Kaveh preferred not to complete the self-report version of the BASC-3, noting he doesn't like to answer so many questions about himself. To maintain rapport, Kaveh was gently encouraged, but the counselor also noted he has the right to assent. It also was felt that if he was unduly influenced to complete the form despite his objection, the data may be inaccurate.

Intervention Design and Implementation

Intervention efforts focused on Kaveh recognizing signs of anxious arousal, identifying anxious cognition, learning appropriate problem-solving strategies and coping skills to manage his frustration, and evaluating himself more positively when experiencing situations that could potentially lead to anxiousness. In reviewing interviews, observations, and assessment data, the counselor hypothesized that Kaveh was engaging in some all-or-nothing thinking, "should" thinking, and catastrophizing. Because Kaveh has a high opinion of himself and is an independent thinker, Socratic questioning techniques would be part of the counseling plan.

Counseling was conducted for 6 weeks, 1 hour per week. Sessions were semistructured such that specific exercises and activities were implemented in a specific sequence while still allowing flexibility to discuss any issues Kaveh presented to the counselor (an outline of each counseling session can be found at the end of this report). Kaveh appeared to be very responsive to working with the counselor and using various strategies discussed. Also, homework was assigned and reviewed each week that emphasized the material covered during each counseling session. The counselor adhered to a cognitive behavioral orientation and adapted sessions from both Kendall's treatment program for youth with anxiety disorders (Coping Cat; Kendall & Hedtke, 2006) and Stark's treatment program for adolescents with depression (ACTION; Stark et al., 2011).

Kaveh was first taught how to become more aware of his own experiences and recognize signs of anxious arousal. Specifically, Kaveh was taught the relationships between his thoughts, emotions, and behaviors and how changing his self-talk (the degree to which it is positive/negative) will impact how he feels and behaves through the use of both positive and negative examples and a thought/emotional charades activity. Kaveh also learned how to differentiate anxiety from other emotions and identified bodily symptoms (through a figure drawing) associated with his anxiety. Therefore, such physiological signs could be used as cues to engage his coping techniques. Additionally, Kaveh participated in exposure tasks that provoke anxiety to (a) help Kaveh realize that imperfection is manageable and (b) practice the skills he learned outside of session. In building a fear hierarchy, Kaveh indicated five fears: getting an answer wrong in front of others, falling off his skateboard at the park, having others know he does not understand some grammar rules, asking the teacher for help in front of peers, and admitting he forgot his lunch money or pencils. In collaboration with teachers, a series of exposures were established (e.g., asking to borrow a pencil because he forgot his, asking for peer and teacher help, letting others see his paper with grammar corrections after it was graded, trying a difficult new skateboard stunt when others were watching, and risking answering in class). Subjective Units of Distress Scale (SUDS) ratings from 1 (no anxiety) to 10 (maximally anxious) were taken during exposures to monitor level of discomfort.

The counselor also sought to identify Kaveh's anxious cognitions and to change negative and self-derogatory thinking to more positive and realistic thoughts. The inflexible core belief at the center of Kaveh's anxiety is that he has to be perfect in every situation; specifically, he notes, "I should do everything right all the time, and I should always be perfect." The counselor worked with Kaveh to evaluate the evidence for that expectation. In doing so, Kaveh identified how his self-talk can include negative self-evaluations, perfect standards for performance, fear of failure, and concern about what others might think. Also, at times his thoughts can be catastrophizing and ruminate out of control. For example, in regard to doing poorly on an academic task, Kaveh indicated the following thoughts: "I'm stupid," "I don't deserve to be in this grade," "I should be held back," and "I feel horrible—my life's never going to be good." Therefore, the counselor worked with Kaveh to restructure his cognition through Socratic questioning to dispel the accuracy of many of his thoughts. Specifically, Kaveh was asked to provide supportive evidence for/against having a specific negative thought and how he could think about and interpret the situation differently (also, this was modeled for Kaveh by the counselor). This provided Kaveh the opportunity to generate alternative positive thoughts that are more realistic and less negative, thus changing his perceptions regarding the potential severity of a situation (e.g., doing poorly on an academic task).

Kaveh also learned how to evaluate himself more accurately and reasonably. Specifically, Kaveh was shown how he could rate himself based on his effort and not the outcome. Also, for challenging tasks, perfect execution should not be expected; therefore, he grew accustomed to rewarding himself for partial success. In addition, given that everyone makes mistakes/forgets, Kaveh learned to accept that he is no exception and should not hold himself to an impossible standard. Since situations will at times be challenging, Kaveh was provided modeling/practice in identifying the positive things he liked about how he handled a situation as well as discussing what he could do differently if the situation were to occur again. Also, Kaveh created a "self-map" indicating several positive attributes about himself that would remain stable regardless of his academic performance.

Another counseling goal was to help Kaveh use problem-solving skills to cope with novel anxiety-provoking situations. In doing so, he identified specific situations and was guided in generating a useable list of coping strategies (e.g., create an exposure or challenge his thoughts). Importantly, his ineffective coping mechanisms were also discussed (e.g., banging head on wall, crawling under the desk, negative self-talk) and replaced with more effective strategies (e.g., taking a break, seeking support, thinking about the situation differently). Lastly, two booster sessions were provided for Kaveh (at 2 and 4 months postintervention) to review strategies and his progress.

Evaluation and Outcome of the Intervention

Pre- and postintervention rating scale data were collected from Kaveh's teacher and his parents. They rated Kaveh's behavior using the anxiety and depression subscales of the BASC-3 at preintervention and 6 months postintervention. Overall, their ratings of both anxiety and depression were lower following the counseling intervention with booster sessions (Figure 1.2). Additionally, Kaveh practiced his exposures over a 3-week period and was able to bring the anxiety SUDS scores elicited by each of them down to a 5/10 or lower. He also reported less avoidance behavior in anxiety-provoking situations. Additionally, no classroom behavioral referrals were noted during the counseling intervention or 6 months postintervention.

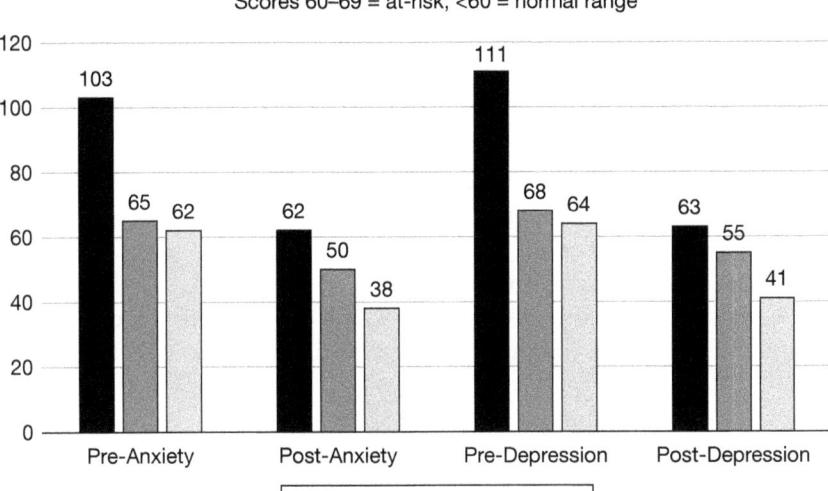

Figure 1.2 Pre- and 6-Months Post-Intervention BASC-3 Data

Counseling Outline

Session 1: Affective Education/Recognize Signs of Anxious Arousal

- Confidentiality, assent, rapport building (Note: Guidelines are discussed in Chapter 3 of this text)
- Become more aware of own feelings before they escalate, physiological cues
- Relationship between thoughts, emotions, and behaviors (Note: The CBT triad is reviewed in Chapter 6 of this text)
- Differentiate anxiety from other emotions
- Identify negative self-talk statements (e.g., "I am stupid")
- Homework: diary of feelings (antecedent, physiological cues, label feeling)

Session 2: Exposure Tasks (Note: The exposure/response prevention technique is discussed in Chapter 7 of this text)

- Build fear hierarchy
- In-vivo exposure (model, utilize coping skills) with SUDS ratings
- Normalize anxiety; it's a manageable experience
- Homework: practice at-home exposures (e.g., new skate park feat in front of others)

Session 3: Identify Anxious Cognition/Cognitive Restructuring (Note: Techniques for challenging cognitive distortions are discussed in Chapter 6 of this text)

- Practice exposures
- Identify inflexible core beliefs (i.e., distortions, all-or-nothing thinking, "should" thinking, catastrophizing)
- Challenging negative self-thought
  - What's another way to think about it?
  - Where's the evidence?
  - Generate alternative positive thoughts
- Homework: list of anxious negative self-talk (generate positive coping self-talk); continue exposure practice at home

Session 4: Develop Coping Skills/Problem Solving

- Practice exposures
- Identify specific situations/settings that are problematic
- Teach problem-solving process (provide examples of situations, help generate alternatives, evaluate possibilities, choose solution)
  - What is the problem?
  - What are all the things I could do about it (brainstorm)?
  - What will probably happen if I do those things?
  - Which solution do I think will work best?
  - After I tried it, how did I do?
- Homework: generate actions to cope from previous list of negative/positive self-talk; continue exposure practice at home

Session 5: Contingency Management/Build Positive Sense of Self

- Practice exposures
- Evaluate own actions more accurately, reasonably, positively
- Teach to rate himself based on effort and not outcome (give examples)
- For challenging tasks, perfect execution is not expected; reward partial success
- Learn to identify things he liked about how he handled the situation and what he would do differently
- Generate list of positive self-rewards
- Homework: interview others, asking how they would evaluate you if you . . .; diary: create list of behaviors that show it is OK not to be perfect

Session 6: Review and Closure (Note: Techniques for terminating therapy are discussed in Chapter 9 of this text)

- Review information from sessions 1 through 5
- Celebrate successes

- Rehearse go-to strategies when anxious
- Provide contact process for school if need more sessions

CHAPTER DISCUSSION QUESTIONS

1. What mental health syndromes are most prevalent in youth?
2. How might counseling services fit within an MTSS model of service delivery?
3. What are some of the similarities and differences between Section 504 plans and IEPs?
4. What special considerations might be pertinent when counseling students with chronic health needs?
5. How do students qualify for special education?
6. What is the difference between ED and OHI classifications?
7. What are some of the benefits of school-based counseling?

REFERENCES

Achenbach, T. M., & Rescorla, L. A. (2001). *Manual for the ASEBA school-age forms & profiles*. University of Vermont, Research Center for Children, Youth, & Families.American Academy of Pediatrics. (2004). Policy statement: School-based mental health services. *Pediatrics*, 113(6), 1839–1844.

American Psychiatric Association. (2013). *Diagnostic and statistical manual of mental disorders* (5th ed.). Author.

Americans with Disabilities Act Amendment Act of 2008, Pub. L. No 110-325, Stat. 3406 (110th) (2008).

Americans with Disabilities Act of 1990, Pub. L. No. 101-336, 104 Stat. 328 (1990).

Atkins, M. S., Hoagwood, K. E., Kutash, K., & Seidman, E. (2010). Toward the integration of education and mental health in schools. *Administration and Policy in Mental Health and Mental Health Services Research*, 37(1–2), 40–47. doi:10.1007/s10488-010-0299-7

Benner, G. J., Kutash, K., Nelson, J. R., & Fisher, M. B. (2013). Closing the achievement gap of youth with emotional and behavioral disorders through multi-tiered systems of support. *Education and Treatment of Children*, 36(3), 15–29. https://doi.org/10.1353/etc.2013.0018

Blanco, C., Bragdon, L. B., Schneier, F. R., & Liebowitz, M. R. (2013). The evidence-based pharmacotherapy of social anxiety disorder. *International Journal of Neuropsychopharmacology*, 16(01), 235–249.

Boekaerts, M., & Roder, I. (1999). Stress, coping, and adjustment in children with a chronic disease: A review of the literature. *Disability and Rehabilitation*, 21, 311–337. https://doi.org/10.1080/096382899297576

Burns, B. J., Costello, E. J., Angold, A., Tweed, D., Stangle, D., Farmer, E. M. Z., & Erkanli, A. (1995). Children's mental health service use across service sectors. *Health Affairs*, 14(3), 149–159.

Canton, J., Scott, K. M., & Glue, P. (2012). Optimal treatment of social phobia: Systematic review and meta-analysis. *Neuropsychiatric Disease and Treatment, 8*, 203–215.

Carpenter, J. K., Andrews, L. A., Witcraft, S. M., Powers, M. B., Smits, J. A. J., & Hofmann, S. G. (2018). Cognitive behavioral therapy for anxiety and related disorders: A meta-analysis of randomized placebo-controlled trials. *Depression and Anxiety, 35*(6), 502–515. https://doi.org/10.1002/da.22728

Centers for Disease Control and Prevention. (2017). *Suicide among youth.* https://www.cdc.gov/healthcommunication/

Clark, E., Russman, S., & Orme, S. (1999). Traumatic brain injury: Effects on school functioning and intervention strategies. *School Psychology Review, 28*, 242–250.

Costello, E. J., Copeland, W., & Angold, A. (2011). Trends in psychopathology across the adolescent years: What changes when children become adolescents, and when adolescents become adults? *Journal of Child Psychology and Psychiatry, and Allied Disciplines, 52*(10), 1015–1025. https://doi.org/10.1111/j.1469-7610.2011.02446.x

Costello, E. J., Copeland, W., & Angold, A. (2016). The Great Smoky Mountains Study: Developmental epidemiology in the southeastern United States. *Social Psychiatry and Psychiatric Epidemiology, 51*(5), 639–646. https://doi.org/10.1007/s00127-015-1168-1

Costello, E. J., Egger, H., & Angold, A. (2005). 10-year research update review: The epidemiology of child and adolescent psychiatric disorders: I. Methods and public health burden. *Journal of the American Academy of Child and Adolescent Psychiatry, 44*(10), 972–986. https://doi.org/10.1097/01.chi.0000172552.41596.6f

Crump, C., Rivera, D., London, R., Landau, M., Erlendson, B., & Rodriguez, E. (2013). Chronic health conditions and school performance among children and youth. *Annals of Epidemiology, 23*(4), 179–184. https://doi.org/10.1016/j.annepidem.2013.01.001

Cuijpers, P., Hollon, S. D., van Straten, A., Bockting, C., Berking, M., & Andersson, G. (2013). Does cognitive behaviour therapy have an enduring effect that is superior to keeping patients on continuation pharmacotherapy? A meta-analysis. *British Medical Journal Open, 3*, Article e002542. http://dx.doi.org/10.1136/bmjopen-2012-002542

Cuijpers, P., Sijbrandij, M., Koole, S. L., Andersson, G., Beekman, A. T., & Reynolds, C. F. (2014). Adding psychotherapy to antidepressant medication in depression and anxiety disorders: A meta-analysis. *World Psychiatry, 13*(1), 56–67. https://doi.org/10.1002/wps.20089

de Gage, S. B., Bégaud, B., Bazin, F., Verdoux, H., Dartigues, J. F., Pérès, K., Kurth, T., & Pariente, A. (2012). Benzodiazepine use and risk of dementia: Prospective population based study. *British Medical Journal, 345*, Article e6231. https://doi.org/10.1136/bmj.e6231

Eagle, J. W., Dowd-Eagle, S. E., Snyder, A., & Holtzman, E. G. (2014). Implementing a multi-tiered system of support (MTSS): Collaboration between school psychologists and administrators to promote systems-level change. *Journal of Educational and Psychological Consultation, 25*(2–3), 160–177. https://doi.org10.1080/10474412.2014.929960

Fixsen, D. L., Naoom, S. F., Blasé, K. A., Friedman, R. M., & Wallace, F. (2005). Implementation research: A synthesis of the literature. https://nirn.fpg.unc.edu/sites/nirn.fpg.unc.edu/files/resources/

Friedberg, R. D., McClure, J. M., & Garcia, J. H. (2009). *Cognitive therapy techniques for children and adolescents*. Guilford Press.

Ginsburg, G. S., Becker, K. D., Kingery, J. N., & Nichols, T. (2008). Transporting CBT for childhood anxiety disorders into inner-city school-based mental health clinics. *Cognitive and Behavioral Practice, 15*, 148–158. https://doi.org/10.1016/j.cbpra.2007.07.001

Gore, F., Bloem, P., Patton, G. C., Ferguson, B. J., Coffey, C., Sawyer, S. M., & Mathers, C. M. (2011). Global burden of disease in young people age 10–24 years: A systematic analysis. *Lancet, 377*, 2093–2102. https://doi.org/10.1016/S0140-6736(11)60512-6

Grapin, S., Waldron, N., & Joyce-Beaulieu, D. (2019). Longitudinal effects of RtI implementation on reading achievement outcomes. *Psychology in the Schools, 56*(2), 242–254. doi:10.1002/pits.22222

Greene, J. P., & Winters, M. (2005). *Public high school graduation and college readiness: 1991–2002*. Manhattan Institute for Policy Research.

Hoagwood, K., & Erwin, H. D. (1997). Effectiveness of school-based mental health services for children: A 10-year research review. *Journal of Child and Family Studies, 6*, 435–451.

Hofmann, S. G., Asnaani, A., Vonk, I. J., Sawyer, A. T., & Fang, A. (2012). The efficacy of cognitive behavioral therapy: A review of meta-analyses. *Cognitive Therapy & Research, 36*(5), 427–440. http://dx.doi.org/10.1007/s10608-012-9476-1

Holler, R. A., & Zirkel, P. A. (2008). Section 504 and public schools: A national survey concerning "Section 504-only" students. *National Association of Secondary School Principals Bulletin, 92*(1), 19–43. https://doi.org/10.1177/0192636508314106

Individuals with Disabilities Education Act of 1990, Pub. L. No. 101-476, 20 U.S.C. §1400 et seq.

Individuals with Disabilities Education Improvement Act of 2004, Pub. L. No. 108-446, 20 U.S.C. §1400 et seq.

Joyce-Beaulieu, D., & Zaboski, B. (2021). Raising the emotional wellbeing of students with anxiety and depression. In P. Lazarus, S. Suldo, & B. Doll (Eds.), *Fostering the emotional well-being of our youth: A school-based approach*. Oxford University Press.

Karpiak, C. P., & Zaboski, B. A. (2013). Lifetime prevalence of mental disorders in the general population. In G. P. Koocher, J. C. Norcross, & B. A. Greene (Eds.), *Psychologists' desk reference* (3rd ed., pp. 3–16). Oxford University Press.

Kendall, P. C., & Hedtke, K. (2006). *Cognitive-behavioral therapy for anxious children: Therapist manual* (3rd ed.). Workbook Publishing.

Kessler, R. C., Berglund, P., Demler, O., Jin, R., Merikangas, K. R., & Walters, E. E. (2005). Lifetime prevalence and age-of-onset distributions of DSM-IV disorders in the National Comorbidity Survey Replication. *Archives of General Psychiatry, 62*(6), 593–602.

Masia Warner, C., Fisher, P. H., Shrout, P. E., Rathor, S., & Klein, R. G. (2007). Treating adolescents with social anxiety disorder in school: An attention control trial. *Journal of Child Psychology and Psychiatry, 48*(7), 676–686. https://doi.org/10.1111/j.1469-7610.2007.01737.x

Masia Warner, C., Klein, R. G., Dent, H. C., Fisher, P. H., Alvir, J., Albano, A. M., & Guardino, M. (2005). School-based intervention for adolescents with social anxiety disorder: Results of a controlled study. *Journal of Abnormal Child Psychology, 33*, 707–722. https://doi.org/10.1007/s10802-005-7649-z

Maslow, G. R., Haydon, A., McRee, A. L., Ford, C. A., & Halpern, C. T. (2011). Growing up with a chronic illness: Social success, educational/vocational distress. *Journal of Adolescent Health*, 49(2), 206–212. https://doi.org/10.1016/j.jadohealth.2010.12.001

McDougall, J., King, G., De Wit, D. J., Miller, L. T., Hong, S., Offord, D. R., Laporta, J., & Meyer, K. (2004). Chronic physical health conditions and disability among Canadian school-aged children: A national profile. *Disability and Rehabilitation*, 26(1), 35–45. https://doi.org/10.1080/09638280410001645076

Merikangas, K. R., Calkins, M. E., Burstein, M., He, J. P., Chiavacci, R., Lateef, T., Ruparel, K., Gur, R. C., Lehner, T., Hakonarson, H., & Gur, R. E. (2015). Comorbidity of physical and mental disorders in the neurodevelopmental genomics cohort study. *Pediatrics*, 135(4), e927–e938. https://doi.org/10.1542/peds.2014-1444

Merikangas, K. R., He, J. P., Burstein, M., Swanson, S. A., Avenevoli, S., Cui, L., Beniet, C., Georgiades, K., & Swendsen, J. (2010). Lifetime prevalence of mental disorders in U.S. adolescents: Results from the National Comorbidity Survey Replication-Adolescent Supplement (NCS-A). *Journal of the American Academy of Child & Adolescent Psychiatry*, 49, 980–989. https://doi.org/10.1016/j.jaac.2010.05.017

Michael, K. D., Albright, A., Jameson, J. P., Sale, R., Massey, C., Kirk, A., & Egan, T. (2013). Does cognitive behavioral therapy in the context of a rural school mental health program have an impact on academic outcomes? *Advances in School Mental Health Promotion*, 6, 247–262.

Mokkink, L. B., Van der Lee, J. H., Grootenhuis, M. A., Offringa, M., & Heymans, H. S. (2008). Defining chronic diseases and health conditions in childhood (0–18 years of age): National consensus in the Netherlands. *European Journal of Pediatrics*, 167(12), 1441–1447. https://doi.org/10.1007/s00431-008-0697-y

Mychailyszyn, M. P., Beidas, R. S., Benjamin, C. L., Edmunds, J. M., Podell, J. L., Cohen, J. S., & Kendall, P. C. (2011). Assessing and treating child anxiety in schools. *Psychology in the Schools*, 48, 223–232. https://doi.org/10.1002/pits.20548

National Association of State Directors of Special Education. (2008a). *Response-to-intervention: Blueprint for implementation—district level*. Author.

National Association of State Directors of Special Education. (2008b). *Response-to-intervention: Blueprint for implementation—school building level*. Author.

National Center for Education Statistics. (2020). *The condition of education*. https://nces.ed.gov/programs/coe/indicator_cgg.asp

Neil, A. L., & Christensen, H. (2009). Efficacy and effectiveness of school-based prevention and early intervention programs for anxiety. *Clinical Psychology Review*, 29, 208–215. https://doi.org/10.1016/j.cpr.2009.01.002

Office of Special Education and Rehabilitative Services, U.S. Department of Education. (2000). *A guide to the individualized education program*. https://www2.ed.gov/parents/needs/speced/iepguide/iepguide.pdf

Parasuraman, S. R., Anglin, T. M., McLellan, S. E., Riley, C., & Mann, M. Y. (2018). Health care utilization and unmet need among youth with special health care needs. *Journal of Adolescent Health*, 63(4), 435–444. https://doi.org/10.1016/j.jadohealth.2018.03.020

Parker, J., Zaboski, B., & Joyce-Beaulieu, D. (2016). School-based cognitive-behavioral therapy for an adolescent presenting with ADHD and explosive anger: A case study. *Contemporary School Psychology*, 20(4), 356–369. doi:10.1007/s40688-016-0093-y

Pinquart, M., & Shen, Y. (2011). Behavior problems in children and adolescents with chronic physical illness: A meta-analysis. *Journal of Pediatric Psychology, 36*(9), 1003–1016. https://doi.org/10.1093/jpepsy/jsr042

President's New Freedom Commission on Mental Health. (2003). *Achieving the promise: Transforming mental health care in America*. Final report (DHHS Publication No. SMA-03-3832). U.S. Department of Health and Human Services.

Rehabilitation Act of 1973. Pub. L. No. 93-112.

Reuben, C. A., & Pastor, P. N. (2013). The effect of special health care needs and health status on school functioning. *Disability and Health Journal, 6*(4), 325–332. https://doi.org/10.1016/j.dhjo.2013.03.003

Reynolds, C. R., & Kamphaus, R. W. (2015). *Behavior Assessment System for Children* (3rd ed.) [Assessment instrument]. Pearson.

Rones, M., & Hoagwood, K. (2000). School-based mental health services: A research review. *Clinical Child & Family Psychology Review, 3*(4), 223–241.

Shaw, S. R., & McCabe, P. C. (2008). Hospital-to-school transition for children with chronic illness: Meeting the new challenges of an evolving health care system. *Psychology in the Schools, 45*, 74–87. https://doi.org/10.1002/pits.20280

Shiu, S. (2001). Issues in the education for students with chronic illness. *International Journal of Disability, Development, and Education, 48*, 269–281. https://doi.org/10.1080/10349120120073412

Silverman, W. K., Ortiz, C. D., Viswesvaran, C., Burns, B. J., Kolko, D. J., Putnam, F. W., & Amaya-Jackson, L. (2008). Evidence-based psychosocial treatments for children and adolescents exposed to traumatic events. *Journal of Clinical Child and Adolescent Psychology, 37*, 156–183. https://doi.org/10.1080/15374410701818293

Sprague, J. (2007). *RtI and behavior support: Yes we have to do it here too!* Retrieved on April 2, 2020, from http://maase.pbworks.com/f/RtI_PBS_Sprague_Apr07.pdf

Stark, K. D., Streusand, W., Arora, P., & Patel, P. (2011). Childhood depression: The ACTION treatment program. In P. C. Kendall (Ed.), *Child and adolescent therapy* (4th ed., pp. 190–233). Guilford Press.

Stoep, A. V., Weiss, N. S., Kuo, E. S., Cheney, D., & Cohen, P. (2003). What proportion of failure to complete secondary school in the US population is attributable to adolescent psychiatric disorder? *Journal of Behavioral Health Services & Research, 30*(1), 119–124. https://doi.org/10.1007/BF02287817

Sulkowski, M., & Joyce-Beaulieu, D. (2014). School-based service delivery for homeless students: Relevant laws and overcoming access barriers. *American Journal of Orthopsychiatry, 84*(6), 711–719. doi:10.1037/ort0000033

Sulkowski, M. L., Joyce, D. K., & Storch, E. A. (2011). Treating childhood anxiety in schools: Service delivery in a response-to-intervention paradigm. *Journal of Child and Family Studies, 21*, 938–947. doi:10.1007/s10826-011-9553-1

U.S. Department of Education, Office of Civil Rights. (n.d.). *Protecting students with disabilities*. https://www2.ed.gov/about/offices/list/ocr/504faq.html

U.S. Department of Health and Human Services. (2000). *Report of the Surgeon General's conference on children's mental health: A national action agenda*. National Institute of Mental Health, Office of Communications and Public Liaison.

U.S. Department of Health and Human Services. (2007). *The national survey of children with special health care needs chartbook 2005–2006*. Health Resources and Services Administration, Maternal and Child Health Bureau.

Wexler, D. (2017). School-based multi-tiered systems of support (MTSS): An introduction to MTSS for neuropsychologists. *Applied Neuropsychology: Child, 7*(4), 306–316. https://doi.org/10.1080/21622965.2017.1331848

World Health Organization. (2001). *World Health Organization report 2001.* https://www.who.int/whr/2001/chapter3/en/index3.html

Zaboski, B. A., Joyce-Beaulieu, D., Kranzler, J. H., McNamara, J. P., Gayle, C., & MacInnes, J. (2019). Group exposure and response prevention for college students with social anxiety: A randomized clinical trial. *Journal of Clinical Psychology, 75,* 1–19. https://doi.org/10.1002/jclp.22792

Zaboski, B. A., Schrack, A. P., Joyce-Beaulieu, D., & MacInnes, J. W. (2017). Broadening our understanding of evidence-based practice: Effective and discredited interventions. *Contemporary School Psychology, 21,* 287–297. https://doi.org/10.1007/s40688-017-0131-4

Zaboski, B. A., & Storch, E. A. (2018). Comorbid autism spectrum disorder and anxiety disorders: A brief review. *Future Neurology, 13,* 31–37. https://doi.org/10.2217/fnl-2017-0030

2

Theory and Research

BRIAN A. ZABOSKI, EMMA ROMAKER, AND
DIANA JOYCE-BEAULIEU ■

HISTORICAL DEVELOPMENT OF COGNITIVE BEHAVIORAL THERAPY (CBT)

CBT dates back at least 70 years to Albert Ellis and Aaron Beck, both dissatisfied with the two prevailing theories: psychoanalysis and behaviorism (Prochaska & Norcross, 2018). Psychoanalysis proposed that human behavior and cognitions are motivated by unconscious instincts and defense mechanisms that shape childhood experiences, which impact adult psychological development (Strachey, 1957). Although Freud's contemporaries modified his original theory, their schools of thought generally focused on revealing and modifying the unconscious to relieve distress (Huprich, 2009). Despite its notoriety, Freud and the psychoanalysts faced a compendium of criticism, including falsifying data, relying on clinical observation, and covertly revising their theory to avoid objections (Cioffi, 1998). Steeped in a tradition of clinical interpretation and judgment, even modern psychoanalysts continue to resist some widely accepted research techniques for establishing treatment efficacy. For example, some believe that "the method of RCTs [randomized clinical trials] is not appropriate for long-term psychodynamic psychotherapy and psychoanalytic therapy lasting several years" (Leichsenring, 2005, p. 844). Consequently, high-quality studies that utilize RCTs are underrepresented in systematic reviews and meta-analyses (de Maat et al., 2013; Smit et al., 2012). This failure over time to build a strong supportive literature base motivated discontent among some early psychoanalysts like Ellis and Beck.

By contrast, the behaviorist paradigm (depending on the specific theorist) emphasized antecedents, stimuli, and consequences in the development and maintenance of behavior (Catania & Laties, 1999). Unlike Freud, John B. Watson (1913), one of the founders of behaviorism, dismissed the study of conscious (and unconscious) phenomena, stating that "psychology must discard all reference to consciousness; when it need no longer delude itself into thinking that it is making mental states the object of observation" (p. 163). Thus, while not outright rejected, thoughts and feelings were absent from behaviorism, since they could not be objectively measured (Skinner, 1974).

Behaviorism also was not without detractors. Philosophers questioned behaviorism's philosophical foundations (Lovejoy, 1922), and cognitive scientists like Chomsky (1959) aggressively denounced behaviorism's dismissal of innate phenomena like language acquisition. In short, behaviorists believed in blank slates, while Chomsky contended that some phenomena (like language acquisition) were innate. Chomsky's charge against behaviorism was that it failed to explain language acquisition exclusively through operant conditioning. Even some behaviorists, like Tolman, questioned the dismissal of inner experience, hypothesizing that lab rats used cognitive maps to navigate mazes (1932). Amid this historical background, Ellis and Beck, the "founding fathers" of CBT, developed their respective theories (Matweychuk et al., 2019, p. 47).

THEORIES OF CBT

Scientific theories are developed to explain a family of facts or data that often result from collecting observations and testing hypotheses (Breakwell et al., 2012; for an advanced critique of theory development in psychology, see Meehl, 1978). But theories do more than just unite data points: They can predict future observations (behaviorist theory predicts that variable rates of reinforcement increase the probability of a behavioral response; Drummond & Sauer, 2018), solve real-world problems (e.g., the germ theory of disease suggests that one should wash one's hands to avoid infection; Larson, 1988), and can usually be falsified (i.e., proven wrong; Popper, 1959/2014). Ellis and Beck attempted to explain a collection of observations about human experience by uniting thoughts, feelings, and behaviors into a theoretical framework. They then used their framework to propose interventions for internalizing and externalizing disorders that therapists continue to use today.

In practice, psychological researchers and clinicians use theories to link philosophical concepts to specific assessment and intervention procedures (Herbert et al., 2013). Consider a child who gets out of her seat during class. Behaviorists might start by assessing the child's behaviors, including the consequences that maintain them and their frequency. They would collect data on events that alter the value of those reinforcers (i.e., setting events) and then develop a clinical hypothesis (the child is engaging in this behavior for attention) and a clinical prediction (ignoring the behavior will decrease its occurrence). Real life is of course more complicated than this example, but theories provide an important organizational scheme to help clinicians answer the question, "Where do I start?"

A theory-driven approach to case conceptualization can improve therapy outcomes, provide a reliable guide for conceptualizing and intervening in difficult cases, and advance the science of psychology (Herbert et al., 2013). One nonrandomized study compared the influence of (a) specific theoretical training to (b) no training on the ability of clients to develop coping skills (Strosahl et al., 1998). The authors found that clients whose therapists underwent specific theoretical training were better able to identify life problems, efficiently cope with those problems, accept their reactions to them, and adhere to the treatment model for a longer duration than the clients whose therapists did not receive specific training. Theory also motivates how interventions are delivered when treating anxiety-related disorders. For instance, understanding antecedent conditions, the functions of behaviors, the power of reinforcement schedules, and the moderating influence of dysfunctional cognitions informs therapists about which exposures to conduct and forewarns them of potential treatment barriers (Abramowitz, 2013; also see Chapter 7).

Moreover, theories can generate new interventions. For example, researchers have used perceptual control theory to create transdiagnostic interventions (interventions that address symptoms across multiple disorders) that may be more applicable to a wider range of presenting problems than traditional CBT (Morris et al., 2016). Similarly, applied behavior analysis started as an application of behaviorist principles for hospitalized patients with schizophrenia (Ayllon & Michael, 1959). Accordingly, the American Psychological Association (2005) emphasizes theory in evidence-based practice. As a result, instructors have incorporated theoretical perspectives into graduate training programs (e.g., Bearman et al., 2015).

Albert Ellis

In the 1940s Albert Ellis, a clinical psychologist and psychoanalyst, questioned psychoanalysis's treatment outcomes as well as its claims that childhood events caused adult psychopathology. Ellis believed that a rational approach to therapy was lacking, compelling him to develop rational-emotive therapy (RET). RET had a unique perspective: To reveal and alleviate client distress, a therapist would assess current cognitive processes (as opposed to dreams or childhood events) and directly confront a client's irrational beliefs (Albert Ellis Institute, n.d.). In 1993 Ellis renamed RET to "rational-emotive behavior therapy" (REBT) arguing that it has "always been one of the most behaviorally oriented of the cognitive-behavior therapies ... showing clients how to use imaginal methods of exposing themselves to phobias and anxiety-provoking situations" (Ellis, 1995, p. 87).

Ellis built the foundation of REBT's famous ABC model by rejecting the commonly accepted idea that antecedents (A) lead to consequences (C); in other words, that activating events directly contribute to related consequences, or A → C. For example, if an individual's childhood experiences (A) were less than favorable, traditional psychoanalysts would have expected that child to encounter emotional difficulties in adulthood. Yet this conceptualization may have victimized clients if they believed that adversities *inevitably* caused dysfunction. Thus, Ellis rejected that A → C because it ignored the beliefs one has about an event and how those beliefs shape emotional responses. Thus, Ellis proposed that activating events

(A) lead to beliefs (B) about those events and that those beliefs are what cause emotional/behavioral consequences (C) (Prochaska & Norcross, 2018). Using the ABC model, Ellis believed that for unwanted consequences to change, one must also change the irrational beliefs that preceded them. To do so, Ellis proposed that clients learn to disrupt (D) their irrational beliefs and unrealistic demands. In doing so, clients create an effective new philosophy (E) that is helpful and adaptive in their daily lives. Figure 2.1 provides a schematic of the] ABC model.

Ellis highlighted several kinds of irrational beliefs, including defining preferences as needs, the inability to tolerate certain events, and defining our individual worth on factors external to ourselves. On this last irrational belief, Ellis frequently encouraged clients to accept themselves unconditionally, an early parallel to today's therapies based on mindfulness (see Chapter 5) and acceptance and commitment (Hayes et al., 2012). Ellis thought that the rigid demands placed on oneself and the outcomes of a rigid mindset were characterized by irrational beliefs and dysfunctional attitudes. For example, a rigid demand like "I should always get perfect grades" might be characterized by catastrophizing, or imagining the worst-case scenario ("If I fail, I'll never get into college!"). Moreover, Ellis believed that when preferences and desires morphed into imperative needs, they influenced one's emotional and cognitive processes, causing emotional disturbances. For example, the reasonable *preference* for getting good grades could turn into an irrational *imperative*, "I must get an A." Holding this irrational *imperative* for all grades over time would be nearly impossible to achieve and would likely lead to unwanted consequences (e.g., anxiety).

In REBT, the therapist has a direct, sometimes confrontational role, and the client actively participates in and out of session. "The therapist encourages, persuades, cajoles, and occasionally even insists that the patient engage in some activity . . . which itself will serve as a forceful counterpropaganda agency against the nonsense he believes" (Ellis, 1962, p. 95). The therapist can identify irrational thoughts by exploring inconsistencies between the client's beliefs and actual events. Through challenging and disputing the irrational beliefs, the therapist heightens the client's conscious awareness and encourages unconditional self-acceptance. Meanwhile, the client is active and engaged, working toward therapeutic goals

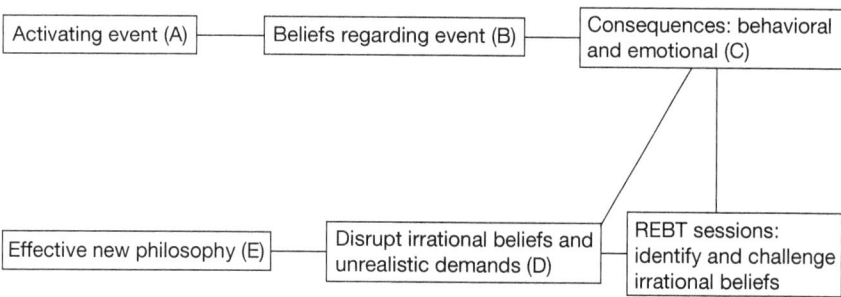

Figure 2.1 The ABC Model

through homework assignments like engaging in a behavioral exposure, logging thoughts, or learning critical thinking skills.

REBT's INFLUENCE

REBT is "the original form and one of the main pillars of cognitive-behavioral therapies" (David et al., 2018, p. 304). REBT shifted psychotherapy dramatically from Freudian approaches that assumed humans are at the mercy of innate instincts and childhood experiences, as well as from behaviorist approaches that dismissed inner experience. Indeed, the REBT approach encouraged therapists to interact and dispute their clients' thoughts to reorient their philosophical worldviews. REBT also used homework, like trying new behaviors and reflecting on one's thoughts. Ellis's work also played an unmistakable role in the development of the ABC model used in a countless number of CBT resources. By the 1980s, REBT became internationally recognized, used in Australia, Europe, Mexico, and Canada (Ruggiero et al., 2014). This widespread usage contributed to REBT applications for new presenting problems, like alcohol and substance use; anxiety; behavioral interventions for children in educational settings (Banks & Zionts, 2009); and marriage/family conflict. Due to its growth, researchers have implemented the REBT framework within basic/fundamental research domains that encourage evidence-based practice (David et al., 2019).

REBT APPLICATIONS

REBT can be applied for intrapersonal, interpersonal, and social problems. Applications for intrapersonal conflict involve interventions for anxiety, self-esteem, and responsibility (Chamberlain & Haaga, 2001; Cristea et al., 2015; Davies, 2006). REBT can be applied to address intimacy/sexual dysfunction, to enhance communication skills, to decrease social hostility, and to reduce a need for interpersonal control (Abrams, 2019; Criddle, 2007). Additionally, it can guide clients through difficult life adjustments and improve impulse control. Aside from treating psychopathology, REBT can also be enhance general wellness, helping clients explore their meaning of life and form their ideal selves.

Some research shows promising outcomes for school-aged children outside of typical therapy sessions. One study tested the efficacy of rational emotive education training for the development of emotional proficiency (Caruso et al., 2018). The rational emotive education preventive program consisted of challenging irrational thoughts, minimizing reaction to frustrating events, and teaching effective coping and self-acceptance practices. The program efficacy was tested on both students (3rd graders) and teachers. The main objectives involved assessing the role of storytelling to decrease irrational thoughts and effects of teacher training on self-efficacy. A positive training effect for students was shown through differences in pre/post training scores on a measure of rational beliefs. For teachers, there was a large difference in pre/post training scores on a measure of self-efficacy ($d = 0.99$), interpreted as an increased ability to manage difficult events and problematic classroom experiences. Overall, these findings suggest beneficial outcomes in classrooms adopting REBT training for both students and teachers.

Aaron Beck

While Ellis published and popularized REBT in the 1950s, Aaron Beck, another trained psychoanalyst, recognized and studied thought patterns among his patients. During free association tasks, a psychoanalytic technique in which patients reveal the unconscious by saying whatever comes to mind, Beck noticed that some of his patients were completely unaware of their thoughts and that their thoughts influenced their affect and behavior. On exploring these thoughts, he also found a cognitive shift among his depressed patients that negatively biased their thoughts about the past, present, and future (Beck, 1976). He named this shift the cognitive triad (sometimes also called the negative triad or triad of depression), and it "has been found across all types and subtypes of depression" (Beck, 1991, p. 372). Figure 2.2 provides a schematic of the cognitive triad model.

Beck also proposed and tested the content specificity hypothesis: Faulty cognitions associated with various disorders are specific to each disorder (Beck et al., 1987). For example, a clinician can expect to observe specific cognitions associated with depression (guilt, shame) and different cognitions for anxiety (threat). The content specificity hypothesis allowed Beck and colleagues to establish maladaptive thoughts common to depressed clients, called depressogenic assumptions. Each assumption is a result of a faulty cognitive process (Prochaska & Norcross, 2018). These common cognitive errors include overgeneralizing, selective abstraction, excessive responsibility, self-reference, and dichotomous thinking (see Chapter 6).

Having made clinical and empirical observations, Beck formulated his cognitive model, heavily influenced by information processing theory (IPT) and Ellis's REBT. At a basic level, IPT proposes that humans do not just mindlessly react to stimuli; rather, they process it first. Beck expanded on IPT, claiming that not only is information processed but also depression and anxiety can bias processing by introducing cognitive errors into one's thinking. These cognitive errors lead to maladaptive beliefs that the mind organizes into larger information structures, called schemas. When activated "by external events, drugs, or endocrine factors, they tend to bias the information processing and produce the typical cognitive content of a specific disorder" (Beck, 2005, p. 954). Consider James, an adolescent who experiences a bad breakup. He might automatically and unknowingly process the event incorrectly, inferring that "It was all my fault, and I'll always be alone." This can then produce maladaptive beliefs ("I'm just not a good boyfriend").

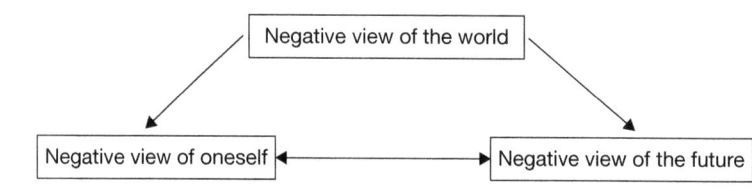

Figure 2.2 Cognitive Triad Model

When these beliefs persist, his mind begins to organize them into larger schemas. When the schema is activated again, like by another guy asking him out, it is accompanied by (a) the belief that he is not a good boyfriend and (b) thinking errors ("There is no point," "Relationships always end in the same way for me") that prevent him from going out on that date.

Thus, Beck's cognitive therapy (CT) approach aims to identify maladaptive, automatic thoughts and directly test them through logic and experiment. It involves three sequential intervention goals:

1. Reduce acute symptoms through contingency management (assigning tasks that reinforce the client's efforts).
2. Evaluate the client's daily activities based on how they impact mood, and assign new contingency management tasks based on this assessment.
3. After problem behaviors improve, explore and challenge the underlying cognitions that contributed to the symptoms. This process encourages distancing: approaching thoughts in an objective manner, reevaluating them, and avoiding blind acceptance of them.

Additionally, CT is known for Socratic dialog, a collaborative strategy that helps adolescents self-discover the maladaptive cognitions that contribute to their emotional distress. This approach encapsulates Beck's idea of "collaborative empiricism," the belief that the therapist and client collaborate to achieve a shared therapeutic mission, rather than a practitioner supplying every answer (Prochaska & Norcross, 2018).

CT's Influence

CT has had a profound impact on the field of psychology. CT contrasts with psychoanalysis's resistance to scientific validation and behaviorism's refusal to recognize inner experience in its models. As Beck tested his theory and assessed his clients, he contributed several assessment tools, including the Beck Depression Inventory-II (BDI-II; Beck et al., 1996), the Beck Anxiety Inventory (BAI; Steer & Beck, 1997), and the Beck Scale for Suicidal Ideation (SSI; Beck et al., 1979). Like Ellis, he created his own institute, which has trained clinicians in CT across the world (Beck Institute, n.d.). CT's strong empirical support has motivated countries to spend hundreds of millions of dollars on intervention programs. It has been the focus of over a dozen meta-analyses corroborating its efficacy and has been tested in hundreds of randomized clinical trials (Hofmann et al., 2013).

CT's Applications

CT has been applied to a wide variety of disorders such as anxiety (Chambless & Gillis, 1993; Clark & Beck, 2011; Forman et al., 2007), depression (Beck, 1979; Dobson, 1989; Young et al., 2014), bipolar disorder (Lam et al., 2010; Newman et al., 2002), personality disorders (Beck et al., 2015; Matusiewicz et al., 2010; Davidson, 2008), and psychotic disorders (e.g., CBT for Psychosis: Hazell et al.,

2016; Morrison & Barratt, 2010). CT has also been applied to posttraumatic stress disorder (Ehlers et al., 2010; Foa & Rothbaum, 1998; Resick et al., 2017), eating disorders (Agras, 2010; Fairburn, 2008), body dysmorphic disorder (Harrison et al., 2016; Wilhelm et al., 2011, 2014), and relational/marital problems (Addis & Jacobson, 1991; Baucom et al., 2008). Given CT's scientific validation, it is reasonable to expect additional applications in the future.

The General Model

Several factors have edged CT's popularity beyond REBT's, though REBT still has some advantages. CT emphasizes empirical findings and therapeutic collaboration (Trower & Jones, 2001). Additionally, it provides a theoretical conceptualization of each disorder, supported by empirical research. CT is rigorously tested, encourages continuous progress monitoring, and can be delivered in either manualized or unstandardized formats. CT also advocates a treatment modality that evolves based on individual client progress monitoring: Practitioners collect data during each session to modify the intervention to a student's unique strengths and struggles (Padesky & Beck, 2003). Moreover, CT's less confrontational (and more Socratic) style may be more appealing to modern practitioners (Ellis, 2001). Nevertheless, Ellis's approach might better address the whole person (rather than just the symptoms), and his writing has been described as more accessible to the layperson (Trower & Jones, 2001). In addition, REBT's ABC model can benefit case conceptualizations: It allows practitioners the flexibility to develop and revise clinical hypotheses throughout the intervention and addresses rigid beliefs early in treatment (Dryden, 2019).

Given the benefits of both approaches, some therapists have advanced a more general model of CBT—conceptualized as a loose relationship between thoughts, feelings, and behaviors—without miring itself in any one theoretical approach. As such, this model is technique focused, incorporating strategies from various domains/schools of thought. For example, a CBT therapist might borrow from the REBT and humanistic perspectives by stressing the present moment (here and now), encouraging active client participation, using a warm and genuine relationship to enhance rapport, and highlighting unconditional self-acceptance. Some researchers believe that this approach emphasizes techniques at the expense of theoretical considerations (Herbert et al., 2013).[1] However, practitioners should remember that because CT is malleably applied to presenting problems, it represents a family of cognitive behavioral approaches, not a single treatment protocol (Hofmann et al., 2013). As such, there is room for a robust theoretical framework *and* for tailoring specific techniques to a client's unique problems. Therefore, we recommend that when practitioners use techniques like some of those described in Chapters 3 and 5, they consider how those techniques advance their intervention goals within their theoretical orientations.

OVERVIEW OF CBT COUNSELING APPLICATIONS

"Internalizing" and "externalizing" are umbrella terms that group problems according to common, maladaptive behaviors. Externalizing problems encompass disorders typically characterized by observably defiant and disorderly conduct (Hinshaw, 1987). Oppositional defiant disorder (ODD), for instance, would fall under externalizing problems. Alternatively, internalizing disorders subsume problems more difficult to observe in students, like depression (Merrell, 2013). CBT has numerous applications for externalizing/internalizing problems, with research groups studying interventions for school- and college-aged students. Most of these approaches use CT or the more general CBT model.

Internalizing Problems

A broad body of research literature establishes CBT as an efficacious intervention for schoolchildren with depression. For example, one meta-analysis aggregated studies on psychological interventions for students with depression. It compared the effects of treatment to a control group response and found a moderate effect size ($d = 0.55$; Cuijpers et al., 2006). Another study randomized high school students to CBT, a supportive control group, or a no-treatment control (Pössel et al., 2013). After a 4-month follow-up, symptom severity in the CBT group was still lower than in the other two groups ($d = 0.29$, $d = 0.30$). CBT's flexibility is also highlighted by a computer-based randomized clinical trial for adolescents in schools conducted by Smith et al. (2015). Compared to a waitlist control, students receiving computer-based CBT evidenced moderate to large improvement on a measure of depression ($d = 0.82$; Smith et al., 2015). These findings support CBT for depression as efficacious and accessible to students in alternative formats.

CBT also addresses anxiety-related disorders in children, adolescents, and college-age students (see Chapter 7). Manassis et al. (2010) conducted a study with elementary and middle school children who screened positive for depression or anxiety and received an after-school group cognitive behavioral intervention versus an active control group. Students in both groups experienced a standard deviation of improvement in anxiety. In another study, researchers randomly assigned African American teens with anxiety to two different group-based interventions: either a school-based CBT group or a supportive control group (Ginsburg & Drake, 2002). Posttreatment, 75% of the students in the CBT group no longer met criteria for an anxiety disorder compared to 20% of students in the control group. Some research also indicates that students use their CBT skills months after treatment ends, supporting evidence for long-term effects. After randomly assigning 7- to 11-year-olds, researchers found moderate effects at a 12-month follow-up for group CBT ($d = 0.65$) and group CBT with parent training ($d = 0.51$) compared to a control (Bernstein et al., 2008).

For college students, researchers investigating the efficacy of CBT with exposure and response prevention also found promising results. For instance, students receiving group CBT with exposure demonstrated moderate improvement on a social anxiety measure even compared to a strong active control ($g = 0.62$; Zaboski et al., 2020). In a meta-analysis of 30 randomized clinical trials using virtual reality exposure therapy for college students, researchers also found large overall effect sizes compared to active controls ($g = 0.78$), with large effects for social anxiety, posttraumatic stress disorder, and panic disorder (Carl et al., 2019). Howell et al. (2019) compared web-based CBT to a control group to investigate whether they could use CBT preventively for graduate students. Controlling for gender and baseline depression, they found small to moderate effects ($d = 0.29$) on anxiety symptom scores. Thus, CBT is efficacious for secondary as well as college students even in well-controlled studies.

Externalizing Problems

Inattention, hyperactivity, working memory deficits, and impulsivity are common among school-aged children, with some youth meeting criteria for attention-deficit/hyperactivity disorder (ADHD). Given the prevalence of ADHD, CBT also has been widely investigated for this population. After a 6-week follow-up, a nonrandomized study of multicomponent CBT for children with ADHD found small improvements for child-reported behavior ($d = 0.10$) and teacher-reported conduct problems ($d = 0.30$); medium improvement for teacher-reported impulsivity ($d = 0.56$); and large improvements on teacher-reported inattention ($d = 1.62$) and hyperactivity ($d = 1.00$; Bloomquist et al., 1991). A meta-analysis with 19 studies on behavioral classroom programs found small decreases in teacher-reported disruptive behaviors ($d = -0.15$), with small to medium effects when measured through classroom observations ($d = -0.48$). Similarly, there were small decreases for teacher-rated ADHD symptoms ($d = -0.19$; Veenman et al., 2018).

For students with more severe behaviors, researchers typically recommend a combined medication and cognitive behavioral intervention strategy (Young & Amarasinghe, 2010), as CBT and pharmacotherapy often synergize. For example, medicated adolescents with ADHD later benefited from CBT, evidenced by large effects on clinician-rated ($d = 0.83$) and parent-rated ($d = 0.79$) symptom severity compared to a waitlist control (Sprich et al., 2016). Child-rated decreases were small ($d = 0.32$). Taken together, these studies show that multimodal cognitive behavioral interventions emphasizing psychoeducation, distraction management, challenging negative thoughts, improving organizational skills, parent training, and teacher consultation may contribute to the effectiveness of CBT.

Autism spectrum disorder (ASD) poses complex challenges that a cognitive behavioral approach also can address, especially for individuals with comorbid anxiety. For instance, research suggests that about 40% of children with ASD have a diagnosed anxiety disorder (Van Steensel et al., 2011), with most children exhibiting social skills deficits, resistance to change, repetitive behavior, and family distress (Zaboski & Storch, 2018). A modified CBT approach considers the child's level of proficiency, incorporates concrete examples, implements behavioral support strategies, avoids abstract discussions, and encourages parent involvement (Rotheram-Fuller & MacMullen, 2011).

An RCT met these challenges (Wood et al., 2009). Using modular and multimodal interventions for children with ASD and anxiety, the researchers integrated social/adaptive skills and attention/motivation training into a CBT protocol that addressed common comorbidities (e.g., anxiety). They found that anxiety disorders remitted in over half of the experimental group. In a separate study, researchers modified Face Your Fears, a group-based CBT intervention, for adolescents in schools with ASD and anxiety (Drmic et al., 2017). The intervention included core CBT principles like psychoeducation, cognitive restructuring, and exposure. They found large pre/post decreases in anxiety ($r = 0.85$), with 44% of children showing anxiety decreases below a clinical threshold. These findings suggest that flexibly delivered, school-based CBT can assist students with comorbid ASD and anxiety.

ODD, conduct disorder, and general behavior problems and defiance can also be addressed through cognitive behavioral interventions. The effectiveness of CBT for externalizing symptoms was reviewed in a meta-analysis that synthesized 21 studies (Battagliese et al., 2015). When tested against control conditions, CBT had a large effect for students with ODD ($d = 0.88$) and externalizing symptoms in general ($d = 0.52$). One popular CBT approach for oppositional and conduct-related problems is the Coping Power Program (CPP), a cognitive behavioral protocol that includes goal setting, academic skill building, recognizing one's cognitive and biological emotional cues, relaxation skills, perspective taking, social problem solving, and resisting peer pressure. Using the CPP for students in two inner-city schools, overall diagnostic risk of ODD, conduct disorder, or ADHD decreased in 60% of students. Moreover, at the conclusion of the intervention, 8% of children no longer met criteria for ODD, and 32% of children had lower ODD symptom severity; there was no meaningful change for conduct disorder.

Even with children exhibiting more severe behaviors, CBT's effectiveness holds. For example, a 6-year outcome study of the CPP in a psychiatric hospital included 9- and 10-year-olds with behavioral disorders (Muratori et al., 2019). Children in the CPP group improved more on a measure of diminished emotionality ($d = 1.25$) than children in a generic multicomponent treatment group ($d = 0.44$). In an earlier study the authors also tested the CPP in schools, with nine classrooms randomly assigned to the CPP or a no-intervention control group (Muratori et al., 2015). The CPP classrooms received 24 sessions of weekly intervention. At the conclusion of the intervention, children in the CPP group mildly improved their prosocial behavior more than the control group ($d = 0.15$). Thus, cognitive behavioral strategies are applicable for a range of impairment, and practitioners can continue those similar strategies in schools.

CASE CONCEPTUALIZATION

Despite their similarities, Ellis and Beck conceptualized cases differently. This section presents a general school-based intervention case and briefly contrasts both approaches. For a deeper understanding of the subtle but important differences between these theories, see Padesky and Beck (2003).

Case Background

Adam is a 14-year-old, White, cisgender male who was referred for counseling to the school social worker by his physics teacher, Mrs. Murray, due to declining grades, irritability, sleepiness in class, and concerning statements (e.g., "Why study? It doesn't matter," "I don't care if I have friends anymore," "I'm just not interested in science anymore"). Mrs. Murray conveyed that after teaching Adam for 2 years, she had never been so concerned. She reported that his self-esteem always seemed a little low compared to his peers', but his grades were generally high in her class and he used to express enthusiasm for the subject material, saying that he wanted to go to college to be a scientist.

The social worker's conversations with other teachers and her thorough records review revealed that Adam lives at home in a middle-class family with his mother, father, and 13-year-old sister, Olivia. Mrs. Murray and two of his other teachers spoke of his family positively and conveyed that they enjoy working with him. When asked about his social life, Mrs. Murray recommended speaking to his math teacher, Mr. Calhoun, who runs the school math club. Mr. Calhoun stated that in math club, Adam used to have a "tight-knit group of friends," but over the past couple of months he seems to have "lost interest." Observations of Adam in the lunchroom indicate that he sits alone silently on one end of the table with his friend group. Of note, Mrs. Murray currently teaches his sister, Olivia, in her life science class, and Olivia told her that Adam is "quiet," "fights with Mom and Dad all the time," and "never leaves his room."

At the conclusion of the first session with Adam, evidence suggests that he has felt more tired recently. He shared that he fights with his parents more and is starting to "hate" them because they "force him" to go to math club, prevent him from napping during the day, and wake him up regularly throughout the week. He is no longer interested in academics and would prefer to stay home and play video games, though he despondently said that they just increase his frustration and that he plays "just to pass the time." Adam said that he has been less involved with his friends because they "just don't get me anymore." Despite these difficulties, Adam has insight that his behavior has changed and admits that he is not happy anymore. Toward the end of the session, he received psychoeducation on depression and was asked if he would like to work on some of his problems. Adam was skeptical that he could improve but agreed to come back. He denied suicidal ideation.

REBT and CBT

Recall the core model of REBT: Activating events (A), such as situations, thoughts, feelings, or behaviors, lead to a belief about the event (B) from which consequences (C) emerge. Beliefs can be rational or irrational, with irrational beliefs more likely to result in maladaptive consequences, like hopelessness, withdrawal, and irritability. Thus, by disputing irrational beliefs (D), Adam will learn an effective new philosophy (E).

By contrast, Beck's CT model for depression challenges dysfunctional cognitions that contribute to the cognitive triad of depression: viewing oneself, the world, and the future negatively. Because these negative thoughts can be automatic, CT advocates that one identify those automatic thoughts and replace them with more adaptive ones.

The goal of REBT is to help Adam create an effective new philosophy, whereas Beck's CT emphasizes challenging cognitive distortions. Both approaches might start by assessing the antecedents, behaviors, and consequences in Adam's life (see Chapters 6 and 7) and then disputing those thoughts, but each approach has a different goal. For example, during your first session, Adam shared that he believes his friends do not understand him anymore. With REBT, you can challenge this by asking, "How helpful is that thought?" "If you did talk to them and they did not understand you, why is that important to your self-worth?" "Does it follow logically that if they do not understand you now, they never could?" Thus, therapists using REBT seek to dispute irrational beliefs to help Adam place a more rational level of importance on his friends' opinions, thereby creating a more effective life philosophy.

Interactions between the therapist and client also differ between approaches. Characteristic of the REBT approach is a confrontational and direct style in which you directly refuting illogical beliefs.

>Adam: My friends will never understand me.
>REBT therapist: They'll *never* understand you or they *might* not understand you?
>Adam: Never, and I need them to understand.
>REBT therapist: You *need* them to? Sounds absolute.
>Adam: Well, I do.
>REBT therapist: That's a strong demand to make of someone, especially since we can't control what they can and cannot understand.
>Adam: Well, I can try.
>REBT therapist: Trying is rational! You can and should try! But when we talk about it as a need, like food or water, we're bound to fail, to be frustrated, and to feel hopeless.

In this dialog, the REBT therapist immediately qualifies an absolute, "never," with a "might." The therapist also highlights Adam's thinking as "absolute" and notes the irrationality of calling it a "need." An error in Adam's philosophical worldview was then examined when the therapist noted that his need for others to understand him cannot always be met. For homework, an REBT therapist might challenge Adam to talk about his thoughts/feelings with his friends to challenge (a) the notion that they will never understand him and (b) the notion that he needs them to.

By contrast, a CT therapist would use Socratic dialogue to help Adam recognize his distorted thought and replace it with something more adaptive:

Adam: My friends will never understand me.
CT therapist: I know that your friends are important to you and so is their understanding. What would you like them to understand?
Adam: I don't know. Maybe what it's like to have depression.
CT therapist: How often do you try to explain this?
Adam: I don't, really. I guess I gave up.
CT therapist: It sounds like on the one hand you want them to understand, but on the other you haven't tried.
Adam: But what if they can't understand me?
CT therapist: Is there any way to know whether they will or not?
Adam: I guess I could try a little harder.

Through Socratic dialogue, the CT therapist helped Adam realize that his isolative behaviors might be exacerbating his distorted thinking. By doing so, the CT therapist can now propose some collaborative experiments in which Adam talks to his friends about his thoughts/feelings and then discusses the outcome with the therapist. Of note, the CT therapist did not explicitly address Adam's philosophical worldview; rather, the goal was to challenge the distorted thinking.

CHAPTER DISCUSSION QUESTIONS

1. One reason behaviorism ignores inner experience is that it cannot be measured. Do you agree that inner experience cannot be measured? Do you agree that if we cannot measure a phenomenon it is not worth considering in our explanations of human behavior?
2. How might REBT or CT be modified for individuals of different racial or ethnic backgrounds?
3. Which therapeutic style do you think is a better match for you, Beck's (Socratic) or Ellis's (confrontational)? Can you think of situations when we might want to use both?
4. Do you agree with Ellis that therapists should be attempting to modify life philosophies, or should therapists focus primarily on maladaptive beliefs as Beck does?
5. While Beck and Ellis famously rejected psychoanalysis for its lackluster treatment outcomes, practitioners around the world continued to

use these methods because they believed them to be effective. Should a similar revolution occur against CBT in favor of a new treatment paradigm?
6. Consider the research presented on internalizing and externalizing problems. Did you notice any weaknesses in the literature?
7. How might developmental considerations complicate the research on CBT?

NOTE

1. Note that this approach differs from psychotherapy integration, an advanced, often empirical/systematic set of approaches for combining techniques across theoretical orientations. See Norcross and Goldfried (2019).

REFERENCES

Abramowitz, J. S. (2013). The practice of exposure therapy: Relevance of cognitive-behavioral theory and extinction theory. *Behavior Therapy, 44*(4), 548–558. https://doi.org/10.1016/j.beth.2013.03.003

Abrams, M. (2019). REBT and sexual problems. In W. Dryden & M. E. Bernard (Eds.), *REBT with diverse client problems and populations* (pp. 127–149). Springer.

Addis, M. E., & Jacobson, N. S. (1991). Integration of cognitive therapy and behavioral marital therapy for depression. *Journal of Psychotherapy Integration, 1*(4), 249–264. https://doi.org/10.1037/h0101197

Agras, W. S. (2010). *The Oxford handbook of eating disorders*. Oxford University Press.

Albert Ellis Institute. (n.d.). *About Albert Ellis, Ph.D.* https://albertellis.org/about-albert-ellis-phd/

American Psychological Association. (2005). Report of the 2005 presidential task force on evidence-based practice. Author. https://www.apa.org/practice/resources/evidence/evidence-based-report.pdf

Ayllon, T., & Michael, J., (1959). The psychiatric nurse as a behavioral engineer. *Journal of the Experimental Analysis of Behavior, 2*(4), 323–334. https://doi.org/10.1901/jeab.1959.2-323

Banks, T., & Zionts, P. (2009). REBT used with children and adolescents who have emotional and behavioral disorders in educational settings: A review of the literature. *Journal of Rational-Emotive & Cognitive-Behavior Therapy, 27*(1), 51–65. https://doi.org/10.1007/s10942-008-0081-x

Battagliese, G., Caccetta, M., Luppino, O. I., Baglioni, C., Cardi, V., Mancini, F., & Buonanno, C. (2015). Cognitive-behavioral therapy for externalizing disorders: A meta-analysis of treatment effectiveness. *Behaviour Research and Therapy, 75*, 60–71. https://doi.org/10.1016/j.brat.2015.10.008

Baucom, D. H., Epstein, N. B., LaTaillade, J. J., & Kirby, J. S. (2008). Cognitive-behavioral couple therapy. In A. S. Gurman (Ed.), *Clinical handbook of couple therapy* (pp. 31–72). Guilford Press.

Bearman, S. K., Wadkins, M., Bailin, A., & Doctoroff, G. (2015). Pre-practicum training in professional psychology to close the research–practice gap: Changing attitudes toward evidence-based practice. *Training and Education in Professional Psychology, 9*(1), 13–20. https://doi.org/10.1037/tep0000052

Beck, A. T. (1976). *Cognitive therapy and the emotional disorders.* International Universities Press.

Beck, A. T. (1979). *Cognitive therapy of depression.* Guilford Press.

Beck, A. T. (1991). Cognitive therapy: A 30-year retrospective. *American Psychologist, 46*, 368–375.

Beck, A. T. (2005). The current state of cognitive therapy: A 40-year retrospective. *Archives of General Psychiatry, 62*(9), 953–959. https://doi.org/10.1001/archpsyc.62.9.953

Beck, A. T., Brown, G., Steer, R. A., Eidelson, J. I., & Riskind, J. H. (1987). Differentiating anxiety and depression: A test of the cognitive content-specificity hypothesis. *Journal of Abnormal Psychology, 96*(3), 179–183. https://doi.org/10.1037//0021-843x.96.3.179

Beck, A. T., Davis, D. D., & Freeman, A. (2015). *Cognitive therapy of personality disorders.* Guilford Publications.

Beck, A. T., Kovacs, M., & Weissman, A. (1979). Assessment of suicidal intention: The Scale for Suicide Ideation. *Journal of Consulting and Clinical Psychology, 47*(2), 343–352. https://doi.org/10.1037//0022-006X.47.2.343

Beck, A. T., Steer, R. A., & Brown, G. K. (1996). *Manual for the Beck Depression Inventory-II.* Psychological Corporation.

Beck Institute. (n.d.). https://beckinstitute.org/

Bernstein, G. A., Bernat, D. H., Victor, A. M., & Layne, A. E. (2008). School-based interventions for anxious children: 3-, 6-, and 12-month follow-ups. *Journal of the American Academy of Child & Adolescent Psychiatry, 47*(9), 1039–1047. https://doi.org/10.1097/CHI.ob013e31817eecco

Bloomquist, M. L., August, G. J., & Ostrander, R. (1991). Effects of a school-based cognitive-behavioral intervention for ADHD children. *Journal of Abnormal Child Psychology, 19*(5), 591–605. https://doi.org/10.1007/BF00925822

Breakwell, G., Smith, J. A., & Wright, D. B. (2012). *Research methods in psychology* (4th ed.). Sage Publications Ltd.

Carl, E., Stein, A. T., Levihn-Coon, A., Pogue, J. R., Rothbaum, B., Emmelkamp, P., Asmudson, G. J. G., Carlbring, P., & Powers, M. B. (2019). Virtual reality exposure therapy for anxiety and related disorders: A meta-analysis of randomized controlled trials. *Journal of Anxiety Disorders, 61*, 27–36. https://doi.org/10.1016/j.janxdis.2018.08.003

Caruso, C., Angelone, L., Abbate, E., Ionni, V., Biondi, C., Di Agostina, C., Mobili, A., Verita, R., Navarra, Ruggiero, G. M., & Mezzaluna, C. (2018). Effects of a REBT based training on children and teachers in primary school. *Journal of Rational-Emotive & Cognitive-Behavior Therapy, 36*, 1–14. https://doi.org/10.1007/s10942-017-0270-6

Catania, A. C., & Laties, V. G. (1999). Pavlov and Skinner: Two lives in science (an introduction to B. F. Skinner's "some responses to the stimulus 'Pavlov'"). *Journal of the Experimental Analysis of Behavior, 72*(3), 455–461. https://doi.org/10.1901/jeab.1999.72-455

Chamberlain, J. M., & Haaga, D. A. F. (2001). Unconditional self-acceptance and psychological health. *Journal of Rational-Emotive & Cognitive-Behavior Therapy, 19*, 163–176. https://doi.org/10.1023/A:1011189416600

Chambless, D. L., & Gillis, M. M. (1993). Cognitive therapy of anxiety disorders. *Journal of Consulting and Clinical Psychology, 61*(2), 248–260. https://doi.org/10.1037/0022-006X.61.2.248

Chomsky, N. (1959). Review of BF Skinner's "Verbal Behavior." *Language*, *35*(1), 26–58.

Cioffi, F. (1998). *Freud and the question of pseudoscience*. Open Court Publishing.

Clark, D. A., & Beck, A. T. (2011). *Cognitive therapy of anxiety disorders: Science and practice*. Guilford Press.

Criddle, W. (2007). Adapting REBT to the world of business. *Journal of Rational-Emotive & Cognitive-Behavior Therapy*, *25*, 87–106. https://doi.org/10.1007/s10942-006-0035-0

Cristea, I. A., Stefan, S., David, O., Mogoase, C., & Dobrean, A. (2015). Rational emotive and cognitive behavior therapy (RE&BT) treatment protocol for anxiety in children and adolescents. In D. David, R. A. DiGuiseppe, & K. A. Doyle (Eds.), *REBT in the treatment of anxiety disorders in children and adults* (pp. 51–66). Springer.

Cuijpers, P., Van Straten, A., Smits, N., & Smit, F. (2006). Screening and early psychological intervention for depression in schools. *European Child & Adolescent Psychiatry*, *15*(5), 300–307. https://doi.org/https://doi.org/10.1007/s00787-006-0537-4

David, D., Cotet, C., Matu, S., Mogoase, C., & Stefan, S. (2018). 50 years of rational-emotive and cognitive-behavioral therapy: A systematic review and meta-analysis. *Journal of Clinical Psychology*, *74*(3), 304–318. https://doi.org/10.1002/jclp.22514

David, D. O., Matu, S. A., Podina, I. R., & Predatu, R. M. (2019). Future research directions for REBT. In W. Dryden & M. E. Bernard (Eds.), *Advances in REBT* (pp. 121–147) Springer.

Davidson, K. (2008). *Cognitive therapy for personality disorders: A guide for clinicians* (2nd ed.). Routledge.

Davies, M. F. (2006). Irrational beliefs and unconditional self-acceptance. I. Correlational evidence linking two key features of REBT. *Journal of Rational-Emotive and Cognitive-Behavior Therapy*, *24*, 113–124. https://doi.org/10.1007/s10942-006-0027-0

de Maat, S., de Jonghe, F., de Kraker, R., Leichsenring, F., Abbass, A., Luyten, P., Barber, J. P., Van, R., & Dekker, J. (2013). The current state of the empirical evidence for psychoanalysis: A meta-analytic approach. *Harvard Review of Psychiatry*, *21*(3), 107–137. https:/doi.org/10.1097/HRP.0b013e318294f5fd

Dobson, K. S. (1989). A meta-analysis of the efficacy of cognitive therapy for depression. *Journal of Consulting and Clinical Psychology*, *57*(3), 414–419. https://doi.org/10.1037/0022-006X.57.3.414

Drmic, I. E., Aljunied, M., & Reaven, J. (2017). Feasibility, acceptability and preliminary treatment outcomes in a school-based CBT intervention program for adolescents with ASD and anxiety in Singapore. *Journal of Autism and Developmental Disorders*, *47*, 3909–3929. https://doi.org/10.1007/s10803-016-3007-y

Drummond, A., & Sauer, J. D. (2018). Video game loot boxes are psychologically akin to gambling. *Nature Human Behaviour*, *2*(8), 530–532. https://doi.org/10.1038/s41562-018-0360-1

Dryden, W. (2019). The distinctive features of rational emotive behavior therapy. In M. E. Bernard & W. Dryden (Eds.), *Advances in REBT: Theory, practice, research, measurement, prevention and promotion* (pp. 23–46). Springer Nature Switzerland AG. https://doi.org/10.1007/978-3-319-93118-0_3

Ehlers, A., Clark, D. M., Hackmann, A., Grey, N., Liness, S., Wild, J., Manley, J., Waddington, L., & McManus, F. (2010). Intensive cognitive therapy for PTSD: A feasibility study. *Behavioural and Cognitive Psychotherapy*, *38*(4), 383–398. https://doi.org/10.1017/S1352465810000214

Ellis, A. (1962). *Reason and emotion in psychotherapy*. Citadel Press.

Ellis, A. (1995). Changing rational-emotive therapy (RET) to rational emotive behavior therapy (REBT). *Journal of Rational-Emotive & Cognitive-Behavior Therapy, 13*(2), 85–89. https://doi.org/10.1007/BF02354453

Ellis, A. (2001). Reasons why rational emotive behavior therapy is relatively neglected in the professional and scientific literature. *Journal of Rational-Emotive and Cognitive-Behavior Therapy, 19*(1), 67–74. https://doi.org/10.1023/A:1007899317618

Fairburn, C. G. (2008). *Cognitive behavior therapy and eating disorders.* Guilford Press.

Foa, E. B., & Rothbaum, B. O. (1998). *Treating the trauma of rape: Cognitive-behavioral therapy for PTSD.* Guilford Press.

Forman, E. M., Herbert, J. D., Moitra, E., Yeomans, P. D., & Geller, P. A. (2007). A randomized controlled effectiveness trial of acceptance and commitment therapy and cognitive therapy for anxiety and depression. *Behavior Modification, 31*(6), 772–799. https://doi.org/10.1177/0145445507302202

Ginsburg, G. S., & Drake, K. L. (2002). School-based treatment for anxious African-American adolescents: A controlled pilot study. *Journal of the American Academy of Child & Adolescent Psychiatry, 41*(7), 768–775. https://doi.org/10.1097/00004583-200207000-00007

Harrison, A., de la Cruz, L. F., Enander, J., Radua, J., & Mataix-Cols, D. (2016). Cognitive-behavioral therapy for body dysmorphic disorder: A systematic review and meta-analysis of randomized controlled trials. *Clinical Psychology Review, 48,* 43–51. https://doi.org/10.1016/j.cpr.2016.05.007

Hayes, S. C, Strosahl, K. D., & Wilson, K. G. (2012). *Acceptance and commitment therapy: The process and practice of mindful change* (2nd ed.). Guilford Press.

Hazell, C. M., Hayward, M., Cavanagh, K., & Strauss, C. (2016). A systematic review and meta-analysis of low intensity CBT for psychosis. *Clinical Psychology Review, 45,* 183–192.

Herbert, J. D., Gaudiano, B. A., & Forman, E. M. (2013). The importance of theory in cognitive behavior therapy: A perspective of contextual behavioral science. *Behavior Therapy, 44*(4), 580–591. https://doi.org/10.1016/j.cpr.2016.03.004

Hinshaw, S. P. (1987). On the distinction between attentional deficits/hyperactivity and conduct problems/aggression in child psychopathology. *Psychological Bulletin, 101*(3), 443–463. https://doi.org/10.1037/0033-2909.101.3.443

Hofmann, S. G., Asmundson, G. J., & Beck, A. T. (2013). The science of cognitive therapy. *Behavior Therapy, 44*(2), 199–212. https://doi.org/10.1016/j.beth.2009.01.007

Howell, A. N., Rheingold, A. A., Uhde, T. W., & Guille, C. (2019). Web-based CBT for the prevention of anxiety symptoms among medical and health science graduate students. *Cognitive Behaviour Therapy, 48*(5), 385–405. https://doi.org/10.1080/16506073.2018.1533575

Huprich, S. K. (2009). *Psychodynamic therapy: Conceptual and empirical foundations.* Taylor & Francis Group, LLC.

Lam, D. H., Jones, S. H., & Hayward, P. (2010). *Cognitive therapy for bipolar disorder: A therapist's guide to concepts, methods and practice* (2nd ed.). John Wiley & Sons.

Larson, E. (1988). A causal link between handwashing and risk of infection? Examination of the evidence. *Infection Control & Hospital Epidemiology, 9*(1), 28–36. https://doi.org/10.1086/645729

Leichsenring, F. (2005). Are psychodynamic and psychoanalytic therapies effective?: A review of empirical data. *International Journal of Psychoanalysis, 86*(3), 841–868. https://doi.org/10.1516/RFEE-LKPN-B7TF-KPDU

Lovejoy, A. O. (1922). The paradox of the thinking behaviorist. *Philosophical Review*, *31*(2), 135–147. http://www.jstor.com/stable/2178913

Manassis, K., Wilansky-Traynor, P., Farzan, N., Kleiman, V., Parker, K., & Sanford, M. (2010). The Feelings Club: Randomized controlled evaluation of school-based CBT for anxious or depressive symptoms. *Depression and Anxiety*, *27*(10), 945–952. https://doi.org/10.1002/da.20724

Matusiewicz, A. K., Hopwood, C. J., Banducci, A. N., & Lejuez, C. W. (2010). The effectiveness of cognitive behavioral therapy for personality disorders. *Psychiatric Clinics*, *33*(3), 657–685. https://doi.org/10.1016/j.psc.2010.04.007

Matweychuk, W., DiGiuseppe, R., & Gulyayeva, O. (2019). A comparison of REBT with other cognitive behavior therapies. In M. E. Bernard & W. Dryden (Eds.), *Advances in REBT: Theory, practice, research, measurement, prevention and promotion* (pp. 47–77). Springer Nature Switzerland AG. https://doi.org/10.1007/978-3-319-93118-0_3

Meehl, P. E. (1978). Theoretical risks and tabular asterisks: Sir Karl, Sir Ronald, and the slow progress of soft psychology. *Journal of Consulting and Clinical Psychology*, *46*(4), 806–834. https://doi.org/10.1037/0022-006X.46.4.806

Merrell, K. W. (2013). *Helping students overcome depression and anxiety: A practical guide* (2nd ed.). Guilford Press.

Morris, L., Mansell, W., & McEvoy, P. (2016). The Take Control course: Conceptual rationale for the development of a transdiagnostic group for common mental health problems. *Frontiers in Psychology*, *7*, 1–15. https://doi.org/10.3389/fpsyg.2016.00099

Morrison, A. P., & Barratt, S. (2010). What are the components of CBT for psychosis? A Delphi study. *Schizophrenia Bulletin*, *36*(1), 136–142. https://doi.org/10.1093/schbul/sbp118

Muratori, P., Bertacchi, I., Giuli, C., Lombardi, L., Bonetti, S., Nocentini, A., Manfredi, A., Polidori, L., Ruglioni, L., Milone, A., & Lochman, J. E. (2015). First adaptation of Coping Power Program as a classroom-based prevention intervention on aggressive behaviors among elementary school children. *Prevention Science*, *16*(3), 432–439. https://doi.org/10.1007/s11121-014-0501-3

Muratori, P., Milone, A., Levantini, V., Ruglioni, L., Lambruschi, F., Pisano, S., Masi, G., & Lochman, J. (2019). Six-year outcome for children with ODD or CD treated with the Coping Power Program. *Psychiatry Research*, *271*, 454–458. https://doi.org/10.1016/j.psychres.2018.12.018

Newman, C. F., Leahy, R. L., Beck, A. T., Reilly-Harrington, N. A., & Gyulai, L. (2002). *Bipolar disorder: A cognitive therapy approach*. American Psychological Association. https://doi.org/10.1037/10442-000

Norcross, J. C., & Goldfried, M. R. (2019). *Handbook of psychotherapy integration* (3rd ed.). Oxford University Press.

Padesky, C. A., & Beck, A. T. (2003). Science and philosophy: Comparison of cognitive therapy and rational emotive behavior therapy. *Journal of Cognitive Psychotherapy*, *17*(3), 211–224. https://doi.org/10.1891/jcop.17.3.211.52536

Popper, K. (1959/2014). *The logic of scientific discovery*. Martino Fine Books.

Pössel, P., Martin, N. C., Garber, J., & Hautzinger, M. (2013). A randomized controlled trial of a cognitive-behavioral program for the prevention of depression in adolescents compared with nonspecific and no-intervention control conditions. *Journal of Counseling Psychology*, *60*(3), 432–438. https://doi.org/10.1037/a0032308

Prochaska, J. O., & Norcross, J. C. (2018). *Systems of psychotherapy: A transtheoretical analysis* (9th ed.). Oxford University Press.

Resick, P. A., Monson, C. M., & Chard, K. M. (2017). *Cognitive processing therapy for PTSD: A comprehensive manual*. Guilford Press.

Rotheram-Fuller, E., & MacMullen, L. (2011). Cognitive-behavioral therapy for children with autism spectrum disorders. *Psychology in the Schools, 48*(3), 263–271. https://doi.org/10.1002/pits.20552

Ruggiero, G. M., Ammendola, E., Caselli, G., & Sassaroli, S. (2014). REBT in Italy: Dissemination and integration with constructivism and metacognition. *Journal of Rational-Emotive & Cognitive-Behavior Therapy, 32*, 183–197. https://doi.org/10.1007/s10942-013-0177-9

Skinner, B. F. (1974). *About behaviorism*. Vintage Books.

Smit, Y., Huibers, M. J., Ioannidis, J. P., van Dyck, R., van Tilburg, W., & Arntz, A. (2012). The effectiveness of long-term psychoanalytic psychotherapy—A meta-analysis of randomized controlled trials. *Clinical Psychology Review, 32*(2), 81–92. https://doi.org/10.1016/j.cpr.2011.11.003

Smith, P., Scott, R., Eshkevari, E., Jatta, F., Leigh, E., Harris, V., Robinson, A., Abeles, P., Proudfoot, J., Verduyn, C., & Yule, W. (2015). Computerised CBT for depressed adolescents: Randomised controlled trial. *Behaviour Research and Therapy, 73*, 104–110. https://doi.org/10.1016/j.brat.2015.07.009

Sprich, S. E., Safren, S. A., Finkelstein, D., Remmert, J. E., & Hammerness, P. (2016). A randomized controlled trial of cognitive behavioral therapy for ADHD in medication-treated adolescents. *Journal of Child Psychology and Psychiatry, 57*(11), 1218–1226. https://doi.org/10.1111/jcpp.12549

Steer, R. A., & Beck, A. T. (1997). Beck Anxiety Inventory. In C. P. Zalaquett & R. J. Wood (Eds.), *Evaluating stress: A book of resources* (pp. 23–40). Scarecrow Education.

Strachey, J. (1957). *The standard edition of the complete psychological works of Sigmund Freud, volume XI (1910): Five lectures on psycho-analysis, Leonardo da Vinci and other works*. Hogarth Press and the Institute of Psycho-analysis.

Strosahl, K. D., Hayes, S. C., Bergan, J., & Romano, P. (1998). Assessing the field effectiveness of acceptance and commitment therapy: An example of the manipulated training research method. *Behavior Therapy, 29*(1), 35–63. https://doi.org/10.1016/S0005-7894(98)80017-8

Tolman, E. C. (1932). *Purposive behavior in animals and men*. University of California Press.

Trower, P., & Jones, J. (2001). How REBT can be less disturbing and remarkably more influential in Britain: A review of views of practitioners and researchers. *Journal of Rational-Emotive and Cognitive-Behavior Therapy, 19*(1), 21–30. https://doi.org/10.1023/A:1007891115800

Van Steensel, F. J., Bögels, S. M., & Perrin, S. (2011). Anxiety disorders in children and adolescents with autistic spectrum disorders: A meta-analysis. *Clinical Child and Family Psychology Review, 14*(3), 302–317. https://doi.org/10.1007/s10567-011-0097-0

Veenman, B., Luman, M., & Oosterlaan, J. (2018). Efficacy of behavioral classroom programs in primary school. A meta-analysis focusing on randomized controlled trials. *PLoS One, 13*(10), 1–23. https://doi.org/10.1371/journal.pone.0201779

Watson, J. B. (1913). Psychology as the behaviorist views it. *Psychological Review, 20*(2), 158–177. https://doi.org/10.1037/h0074428

Wilhelm, S., Phillips, K. A., Didie, E., Buhlmann, U., Greenberg, J. L., Fama, J. M., Keshaviah, A., & Steketee, G. (2014). Modular cognitive-behavioral therapy for body dysmorphic disorder: A randomized controlled trial. *Behavior Therapy, 45*(3), 314–327. https://doi.org/10.1016/j.beth.2013.12.007

Wilhelm, S., Phillips, K. A., Fama, J. M., Greenberg, J. L., & Steketee, G. (2011). Modular cognitive–behavioral therapy for body dysmorphic disorder. *Behavior Therapy, 42*(4), 624–633. https://doi.org/10.1016/j.beth.2011.02.002

Wood, J. J., Drahota, A., Sze, K., Har, K., Chiu, A., & Langer, D. A. (2009). Cognitive behavioral therapy for anxiety in children with autism spectrum disorders: A randomized, controlled trial. *Journal of Child Psychology and Psychiatry, 50*(3), 224–234. https://doi.org/10.1111/j.1469-7610.2008.01948.x

Young, S., & Amarasinghe, J. M. (2010). Practitioner review: Non-pharmacological treatments for ADHD: A lifespan approach. *Journal of Child Psychology and Psychiatry, 51*(2), 116–133. https://doi.org/10.1111/j.1469-7610.2009.02191.x

Young, J. E., Rygh, J. L., Weinberger, A. D., & Beck, A. T. (2014). Cognitive therapy for depression. In D. H. Barlow (Ed.), *Clinical handbook of psychological disorders: A step-by-step treatment manual* (pp. 275–331). Guilford Press.

Zaboski, B. A., Joyce-Beaulieu, D., Kranzler, J. H., McNamara, J. P., Gayle, C., & MacInnes, J. (2020). Group exposure and response prevention for college students with social anxiety: A randomized clinical trial. *Journal of Clinical Psychology, 75*(9), 1489–1507. https://doi.org/10.1002/jclp.22792

Zaboski, B. A., & Storch, E. A. (2018). Comorbid autism spectrum disorder and anxiety disorders: A brief review. *Future Neurology, 13*(1), 31–37. https://doi.org/10.2217/fnl-2017-0030

3

Counseling Preparation

DIANA JOYCE-BEAULIEU AND BRIAN A. ZABOSKI ■

One of the keys to successful counseling is advance planning with thoughtful consideration for ethical and legal guidelines. Prior to the first counseling session, it will be important to consider the referral source. Typically in school systems, counseling referrals are initiated by school personnel or parents. However, students may also self-initiate, or outside health providers like pediatricians, social workers, pastoral counselors, or psychologists might recommend counseling, too. Next, practitioners review the referral information to determine the type of therapy needed, time sequence, and goals. This may include reviews of school performance, attendance, and school medical records.

As noted in Chapter 1, when counseling is required by an Individualized Education Program (IEP), the team documentation will often designate frequency, intensity (i.e., session length), and duration. IEPs also require written goals and measurable outcomes. Thus, selection of progress monitoring methods may be required in preplanning. Yet even in the absence of an IEP, MTSS provisions require school-based practitioners to consider how they will measure a student's progress over time. Additionally, interviews with the student, parents, teachers and any referring outside providers can offer insights into student needs. As an example, parents can provide information on personal stressors, any history of mental health hospitalizations, medications, and concurrent therapy. Outside care providers can collaborate on recommended therapy goals and strategies. In some cases, this collaboration may entail having the school-based counseling reinforce concepts from outside therapy or dividing goals so that the school is addressing school-based needs and the outside therapist is addressing family dynamics. Teachers will have insights on behavioral manifestations of symptoms and the student's peer influences. Together the combination of records review and interview processes will aid in case conceptualization, as described in Chapter 2.

LEGAL GUIDELINES

Understanding state and federal laws that address student records and confidentiality is an essential component of counseling preparation. The two most commonly applicable to counseling in school settings are the Family Educational Rights and Privacy Act (FERPA; 20 U.S.C. § 1232g; 34 CFR Part 99; 1974) and the Health Insurance Portability and Accountability Act of 1996 (HIPAA, Public Law 104-191; 1996). These two provisions require care in accessing and divulging information from students' educational and medical records (respectively) within the legal parameters of the statutes. Generally, school counseling personnel may access information for legitimate educational and therapeutic treatment planning needs but must maintain confidentiality and utilize the information only for the direct provision of services. When social workers, counselors, and psychologists create and submit their own documentation (e.g., counseling summaries or reports) at problem-solving team meetings, it may become part of the student's academic or medical records, so care must be given to comply with both FERPA and HIPAA.

FERPA

FERPA provides federal protection for the privacy of students' educational records. The law applies to all schools receiving funding from the U.S. Department of Education. Therefore, private and religious schools may be exempt (U.S. Department of Health and Human Services [USDHHS] & U.S. Department of Education [USDOE], 2008). Rights are provided to the parents but transfer to the student at the age 18 (known as eligible students). Provisions include parents' rights to inspect, review, and correct their child's records. Additionally, parental or eligible student consent is required for release of records. There are exceptions to the consent rule, including:

- School officials with legitimate educational interest
- Other schools to which a student is transferring
- Specified officials for audit or evaluation purposes
- Appropriate parties in connection with financial aid to a student
- Organizations conducting certain studies for or on behalf of the school
- Accrediting organizations
- Compliance with a judicial order or lawfully issued subpoena
- Appropriate officials in cases of health and safety emergencies
- State and local authorities, within a juvenile justice system, pursuant to specific state law (FERPA, 1974; USDOE, 2020).

HIPAA

HIPAA provides federal protection for the confidentiality of protected health information (PHI) (HIPAA, 1996). PHI includes any identifying information that can be linked to an individual (e.g., name, address, phone number, email address, social security number). HIPAA also requires consent for release of records. Exceptions to the consent rule for healthcare providers include serious wounds (e.g., stab, gunshot, injuries from a crime), infectious disease, and child abuse (Edemekong et al., 2020). These exceptions are especially important for counselors when working with school-based threat assessments, school site crimes, and reporting abuse.

HIPAA applies to covered entities: individuals working in healthcare (including private practice), practica students, and companies involved in insurance, billing, and electronic medical records (HIPAA, 1996). It is important to note that most school-based counselors, social workers, and psychologists are typically direct employees of the school system; however, many also are privately contracted personnel who conjointly work in both healthcare settings and school systems. It would be especially important for these providers to be cognizant of the settings, types of information accessible at each setting, and restrictions on transferring information from one setting to another. Within school systems, PHI is sometimes provided by parents to the school nurse to assist in treatment and medication management, to counseling personnel to help inform intervention planning, and to special education eligibility teams to inform placement criteria and accommodation/modification goals.

Intersection of FERPA and HIPAA

The overlap between FERPA and HIPAA law can be confusing, and there are several situations in which the two laws intersect. As noted previously, counselors in both school districts and healthcare facilities need to be cognizant of their roles and boundaries in each setting. Additionally, when parents consent to have outside healthcare providers share information with school service personnel, this places responsibility for appropriate use and disclosure of the information on school personnel. Parents and guardians also may provide copies of mental health treatment reports containing PHI to schools for educational and intervention planning. If these reports are included in the students' educational records, they become subject to FERPA rules. School nurses also have access to student immunization and health records, but because they are kept at the school they are deemed educational records subject to FERPA (USDHHS & USDOE, 2008). For practitioners working in postsecondary settings, students' medical and treatment records are not considered educational records. Further guidance is available through both the USDHHS and the USDOE (USDOE, 2020; USHHS, 2020; USHHS & USDOE, 2008).

PROFESSIONAL ETHICS CODES

In addition to FERPA and HIPAA, there also are ethical guidelines provided by professional organizations for practitioners engaging in counseling services. Agencies most relevant to school-based services include the American Psychological Association (APA), the National Association of School Psychologists (NASP), the American Counseling Association (ACA), and the National Association of Social Workers (NASW). Their ethical codes cover a wide range of professional conduct issues, including competency, fees, advertising, resolving conflicts, research, supervision, and training. Provisions from these agencies specific to counseling therapy follow.

Consent, Assent, and Confidentiality

The APA Ethical Principles of Psychologists and Code of Conduct provisions include counseling services (APA, 2017). The core principles require discussing confidentiality and the limits to confidentiality with clients at the onset of counseling, with reminders when new circumstances arise. Determining who the actual client is will also be a consideration when working with youth. In many cases the parent or an agency has initiated the counseling and may well be considered the client; thus, consent is solicited from the parent. This is a clearer circumstance in hospital, outpatient, and private practice settings, when the individual paying for and initiating services is the client (Coffman & Barnett, 2015). When working with very young children, it may be unclear if they are capable of understanding consent; thus, consent from the parent and assent (or agreement or understanding) from the child may be preferred. Snyder and Barnett (2006) suggest that four criteria must be met for an individual to be capable of consent: Consent must be given voluntarily, the client must be competent (legally as well as cognitively/emotionally) to give consent, the therapist must be sure that the client understands what is being agreeing to, and information shared must be documented. Following these recommendations, students with diminished cognitive capabilities, with emotional distress, or of a young age may not be capable of truly comprehending consent. Therefore, it will be important to actively assess ability to give consent at the onset of counseling.

The NASP (2020) professional standards and ethical guidelines require seeking *parental consent* and *student assent* prior to counseling (with some noted exceptions). Standard I.1.2, Consent to Establish a School Psychologist–Client Relationship, addresses the client relationship:

> Except for urgent situations or self-referrals by a minor student, school psychologists seek parental consent (or the consent of an adult student) prior to establishing a school psychologist–client relationship for the purpose of psychological diagnosis, assessment of eligibility for special education or disability accommodations, or to provide ongoing individual or group counseling, or other therapeutic intervention outside the classroom. (NASP, 2020, p. 42)

NASP exceptions to gaining parental consent are established in Standards I.1.2a and I.1.2.b:

> I.1.2a It is ethically permissible to provide psychological assistance without parental notice or consent in emergency situations or if there is reason to believe a student may pose a danger to others; is at risk for self-harm; or is in danger of injury, exploitation, or maltreatment. (NASP, 2020, p. 42)

> I.1.2b When a student who is a minor self-refers for assistance, it is ethically permissible to provide psychological assistance without parental notice or consent for one or several meetings to establish the nature and degree of the need for services and to ensure that the child is safe and not in danger. (NASP, 2020, p. 42)

Standard I.1.3 discusses the requirement for discussing confidentiality with the student prior to beginning counseling:

> School psychologists ensure that an individual providing consent for school psychological services is fully informed about the nature and scope of services offered, assessment/intervention goals and procedures, any foreseeable risks, the cost of services to the parent or student (if any), and the benefits that reasonably can be expected. The explanation includes discussion of the limits of confidentiality, who will receive information about assessment or intervention outcomes, and the possible consequences of the assessment/intervention services being offered. (NASP, 2020, pp. 42–43)

Standard I.1.4 addresses *assent* and recommends that students participate in the decision to provide services when possible and provide assent for those services:

> Ordinarily, school psychologists seek the student's assent to services; however, it is ethically permissible to bypass student assent to services if the service is considered to be of direct benefit to the student and/or is required by law. (NASP, 2020, p. 42)

If counseling is delivered through electronic or virtual telehealth modalities, therapists must advise clients of the limits and possible risks to confidentiality via that medium (APA, 2017). Confidentiality in therapy sessions is protected to the greatest extent possible within the parameters of federal law and state legal jurisdictions. Psychologists also are prohibited from disclosing the identity of clients for didactic or other purposes. This provision may be of particular importance to faculty and students learning counseling skills, gathering counseling data for research, and presenting case studies at conferences or in publications. For these types of activities, protection of the clients' identity by disguising both the person and organization is required (APA, 2017, see 4.07 for additional information). In working with K-12 students, it also may be important to consider developmentally appropriate statements for confidentiality. For beginning counseling students, the direct supervisor will provide explicit confidentiality procedures. Here are two examples, one adapted for younger children and one for older students:

1. What you tell me in counseling stays with me, except for three things:
   a. If someone is hurting you,
   b. If you are hurting someone else, or
   c. If you want to hurt yourself.
   If so, I will need to get help from other adults so you can be safe.
2. Our counseling session discussions, notes, and correspondence by phone or email are confidential, with some exceptions:
   a. If a judge provides a court order,
   b. If you are under 18 and indicate someone is abusing you physically or sexually,
   c. If you indicate intention to seriously harm others, or
   d. If you indicate intention to self-harm.
   Depending on the circumstance, I will need to report to child protective service, law enforcement, or the intended victim, or refer for hospitalization.

Abuse and Mandatory Reporting

The Federal Child Abuse Prevention and Treatment Act (CAPTA) requires that every state have mandated reporters when child abuse or neglect is suspected. Although there is variation in the procedures and groups of individuals required to report, most states mandate school personnel, social workers, healthcare workers, counselors, therapists, and law enforcement officers to report (Child Welfare Information Gateway, 2019). These requirements also place responsibility on the institutions to provide procedures and systems that ensure personnel are aware of the mandates and that reporting standards are met. Some communication may be considered privileged and the reporter's identity may be protected from disclosure. Before starting counseling, it will be important for the therapist to know local policies and the state's mandated reporter statutes should the need arise.

Recordkeeping

Documentation of counseling sessions may be as simple as a log with names, times, dates, and session outcomes or more complex notes including a problem statement, discussion points, strategies learned, assessment data, and action items for homework. The simple log approach is often utilized for small-group counseling with a prescribed curriculum or to document service compliance for IEPs. For individualized therapy, the more comprehensive form can help counselors maintain structure in the sessions, track progress monitoring data, monitor action steps and homework, as well as plan for subsequent sessions.

The type of documentation may also be influenced by the purpose and audience for the documentation. As an example, counseling related to court cases (e.g., custody, abuse, neglect) may require both the service provision log summary and information on targeted goals and outcomes set by the referring (sometimes called custodial) agency. Another example might be collaborative counseling with outside providers. This type of documentation will require the service provision components of the log format but may also have explicit school exercises (e.g., exposures for phobias or social anxiety) that promote generalization of skills taught in sessions. Counseling linked to outside providers who are providing medical trials (e.g., psychiatrists) may require specific observations, school records, or behavioral ratings for medication effects. Examples might include time-on-task observations for attention deficits, discipline referrals for conduct problems, or attention rating scale scores.

In considering documentation, it is important to remain cognizant of FERPA and HIPAA privacy provisions regarding how information is identified and who has access to the information. The APA (2007) has provided six guidelines for recordkeeping by psychologists:

1. Psychologists maintain responsibility for retention of their records.
2. Psychologist strive to maintain accurate records including pertinent service documentation (e.g., type of service, progress, delivery dates/times, any fees) appropriate to the circumstances and as required by the psychologist's jurisdiction.
3. Psychologists ensure reasonable steps to maintain confidentiality.
4. Psychologists inform clients of the nature, extent, and limits to confidentiality for records.
5. Psychologists organize and maintain accurate records that others with legitimate access to them will find easy to use.
6. Psychologists takes reasonable steps to protect records from damage or inappropriate use.

Similar guidelines are provided by the ACA (2014; Mitchell, 2007). The ACA ethical code also indicates that counselors do the following:

Maintain records necessary to deliver services
Ensure they are secure for authorized users only
Acquire consent prior to creating any audio or video recordings
Provide copies of documents to clients on request (assuming the client is competent)
Only provide individuals with their portion of session notes if the sessions include multiple persons (e.g., group therapy)

- Assist in interpreting any records provided
- Obtain permission before transferring records to other providers
- Store records of terminated therapy in compliance with the timeframes designated by local jurisdictions
- Give careful consideration to destroying any records that might be needed later for a court case (e.g., abuse, suicide).

GROUP OR INDIVIDUAL CBT CONSIDERATIONS

With an understanding of the ethical and legal issues involved in counseling services, practitioners can decide how to format their sessions to ensure structure and continuity. One of the first decisions may be whether to provide small-group or individual therapy. For school-based referrals, this decision may already be made by a district-wide model (e.g., MTSS procedures) or school-based counseling program (e.g., a stepped-care model). Otherwise, practitioners should judge the level of frequency, intensity, and duration of supports a client needs. Another consideration is how common the need may be within a grade level and if counseling would be efficient in small groups. As an example, school systems typically have clusters of children and adolescents with mild to moderate social anxiety who can benefit from group therapy. Conversely, student needs may be too personal (e.g., trauma) or severe for group therapy.

Numerous studies demonstrate the efficacy of group CBT. In a 3-year study of two K-8, low-income, urban schools, three group CBT programs were provided for students with externalizing, anxiety, or depression needs (Eiraldi et al., 2016). The Coping Power Program (CPP) was provided for externalizing disorders and includes anger management, emotional awareness, and problem-solving skills. The Friends for Life (FRIENDS) program was provided for anxiety and addresses physiological, learning, and cognitive processes that maintain excessive anxiousness. Lastly, the Primary and Secondary Control Enhancement Training (PASCET) was implemented for students with depression and targets engaging in activities to lift mood, skill building, identifying and changing depressive thoughts, relaxation, and cognitive techniques for improving mood. Groups included 3 to 5 students, and all 114 participants were receiving free or subsidized lunch. The sample was overwhelmingly minority (African American and Hispanic), 63% male, and matched for gender and race/ethnicity. When analyzing pretreatment and posttreatment data, researchers found that therapy was effective in reducing diagnostic symptom severity for all three groups.

A meta-analysis of group CBT studies for adolescents with depression also found this form of counseling service delivery effective (Keles & Idsoe, 2018). The researchers reviewed 23 studies and found that group CBT was effective at both postintervention and follow-up stages when compared to inactive control groups. Participants receiving group CBT had better results than control conditions when measured at the end of intervention (standardized mean difference [SMD] = −0.28; 95% confidence interval [CI], −0.36 to −0.19) and also at follow-up (SMD = −0.21; 95% CI, −0.30 to −0.11). It was noted that studies with longer follow-up duration were associated with significant, albeit smaller, effect sizes. Similar results were noted for group CBT studies of adolescents with anxiety (Zhou et al., 2018). Investigators reviewed studies of adolescents under age 18 and compared baseline, treatment outcomes, and follow-up scores on anxiety. Eleven forms of psychotherapy (e.g., group/individual CBT, CBT with family, CBT with bibliotherapy, internet-assisted CBT) across 101 studies were analyzed, and studies included both group and individual counseling formats. Four control conditions were found across studies (waitlist treatment, psychological placebo, no treatment, and treatment as usual). All of the psychotherapy formats were significant when compared to the waitlist groups at posttreatment and follow-up. However, only the CBT group therapy was significantly more effective across all control conditions (SMD = −1.43 to −0.76). The authors concluded that group CBT was the most effective for lowering anxiety symptoms and increasing quality of life.

In a sample of college students, group CBT with exposure response prevention also was found effective in treating anxiety and depression for individuals with social anxiety (Zaboski et al., 2019). The study participants included 31 students randomly assigned to an exposure-only group or an active control and found more than a standard deviation improvement in the intervention group.

THERAPY HOMEWORK

Incorporating targeted homework items into counseling plans offers the opportunity for students to practice strategies, reinforce concepts, and generalize these strategies outside of the therapy session. Examples of therapy homework might include increasing scheduled pleasurable activities for an individual with depression or self-initiated social interactions outside of therapy for a child with social anxiety. Kazantzis et al. (2000) conducted a meta-analysis of 46 cognitive and behavioral therapy studies and compared the studies with homework to those without homework. Although the studies indicated both groups improved from pretreatment to posttreatment, effects were larger for the studies with homework. A meta-analysis 10 years later, including 23 studies with 2,183 participants, also found small to medium positive effects for homework ($r = 0.26$; Mausbach et al., 2010). When comparing effect sizes for therapy with homework by targeted symptoms (i.e., anxiety, depression, or substance use), all were effective ($r = 0.22$ to 0.27).

WHAT ARE MICRO SKILLS?

Successful counseling incorporates basic micro skills that will foster rapport, mutual respect, and trust in a diverse caseload of clients. Often clients are addressing problems that are painful for them to discuss, perhaps embarrassing, and sometimes bewildering. Moreover, some students may not have even self-initiated counseling because parents or school personnel may have referred them. These circumstances require rapport building between the student and therapist to establish open communication and comfort with self-disclosure. Micro skills include communication skills that can ease students into disclosing their thoughts and feelings. These skills are also tools for acquiring client information to improve the efficiency and efficacy of sessions (Daniels & Ivey, 2007; Ivey et al., 2017). This section will review the five basic listening sequence components: client observation, attending, open/closed-ended questions, encouraging/paraphrasing/summarizing, and reflection of feelings (Daniels 2010; Daniels & Ivey, 2007). Many different models of micro skills exist (for additional review of various approaches and historical developments see Egan, 2007; Hill, 2004; Ivey et al., 2017; Truax & Carkhuff, 1967).

Client Observation

Client observation encompasses careful monitoring of students' verbal and nonverbal behaviors to better understand and serve their needs. Noticing their voice tone/quality, word choices (e.g., "I feel down" vs. "I feel devastated"), elaborations, and even silence can provide insight into clients' feelings and thought patterns, as well as their ability to label and express them. For instance, a child who is unable to articulate feelings may benefit from emotional vocabulary building (Santiago-Poventud et al., 2015). A student who appears to be asking for help but unable to talk may need more rapport building, may be suffering from anxiety, or may be generally overwhelmed. Similarly, nonverbal qualities (e.g., withdrawal, body posture, eye contact, shuffled walking, fatigue, profuse sweating, panic) may identify emotional states, mental health symptoms, energy level, and social interaction skills.

Additional observational considerations include congruence and discrepancies. When words and nonverbal expressions are incongruent, it may be important for the therapist to ask additional questions and foster further elaboration to better understand why the behaviors and discussion do not match expressed emotions. As an example, sometimes individuals engage in a nervous form of laughter when stressed that would be incongruent with a serious topic. Verbal or nonverbal cues may also alert counselors that a topic may be particularly sensitive or an area of need.

Attending

Attending requires therapists to monitor themselves for any distracting or invalidating behavior, use verbal tracking techniques, and monitor their nonverbal body language. Examples of therapist distractors might include their own fidgeting, frequently adjusting clothing or posture, responding to extraneous stimuli (e.g., a cellphone), or shuffling objects on the desk. Although minor, these actions can communicate a disinterest in the client and could cause the counselor to miss important nonverbal and verbal cues by being inattentive to the student. Should an unintended interruption occur, it can be handled with the Triple A steps (AAA):

An Acknowledgment, perhaps with an apology for the interruption
An Action step to end the distractor
An Affirmation that the client is the priority (e.g., "I'm sorry they're vacuuming outside; I'll ask them to return later because our time together is important").

Verbal tracking includes astute awareness of the ebb and flow of the therapeutic conversation. From the therapist's initial greeting at the start of the session to summarizing homework goals, the counseling dialog should reflect an interrupted message of support. Examples of verbal content tracking include avoiding going off topic (e.g., "Excuse me, I just noticed the A/C filter in here needs changing"), avoiding abrupt changes of topic (e.g., "So I know we were discussing your trama but let's talk about organization skills now."), and strategically encouraging key discussion points through questions or nonverbal acknowledgment (e.g., nodding one's head). Verbal tracking additionally includes self-monitoring one's tone, rate of speech, and idioms. When possible, match these to those of the client, as such congruence can increase the authenticity of the conversation. At times, the therapist will also need to gently redirect conversations to keep verbal tracking aligned with therapeutic goals.

Supportive body language also improves attending. Good eye contact will include a warm expression without uncomfortably staring at a client. Moreover, effective therapists might lean slightly forward to signal interest, model a relaxed and calm body posture, or use small hand gestures (e.g., open palms). Likewise, a quizzical expression may signal to clients the need to elaborate or clarify. Remember, the ultimate goal of attending is to hear clients and understand their needs. Experienced counselors attend not only to the words clients use but also to the words they do not.

Open/Closed-Ended Questions

Counselors utilize two basic types of questions. Closed-ended questions can be answered with a yes/no or a very short factual response. While these are sometimes necessary (e.g., when asking about suicidal ideation), they do not promote elaboration or foster a deep contextual understanding of the student's experience. By contrast, open-ended questions solicit more information and require an explanation or detailed description. These may permit greater insight into the client's thought process. Here are some examples of open and closed-ended questions a therapist could ask to elicit information on the same topic:

1. Do you think the homework was helpful? (closed, yes/no)
2. What did you think of the homework strategies? (open)
3. Do you know what to say when you talk to your mother? (closed, yes/no)
4. What are some of the things you could say when you talk to your mother? (open)
5. When is the best time to start using your deep breathing relaxation technique? (closed; requires a short factual response like "on the weekend")
6. How can you build the deep breathing relaxation technique into your schedule? (open)

When composing questions, we recommend avoiding leading questions that evoke a specific answer, like "How angry was your father?" (which assumes the client's father was angry). Trying not to narrow response options unnecessarily is another important technique, as in "Is he mad at you or just tired?" (which creates a false dichotomy; the client's father could have been anxious, too). Additionally, long, multifaceted questions or those with obscure language can be confusing (e.g., "The next time you are upset, will you think of what options you have, how you will handle obstacles, and what you expect the potential outcomes to be?"). By asking clear and open-ended questions, therapists encourage introspection and learn more about their clients.

Encouraging/Paraphrasing/Summarizing

Encouraging, paraphrasing, and summarizing are techniques that validate the client's experience, synthesize information, and direct the conversation.

Encouraging may include empathy, praise, acknowledgment of progress, or courageousness when addressing difficulties. For instance, in responding to a student who discusses a traumatic event, a social worker might say, "That must have been incredibly difficult to discuss. I have a huge amount of respect for your bravery."

Paraphrasing translates client discussion into pithy phrases that clarify particular points. For example:

Client: Yesterday after I tripped in the hallway, I went into class and everyone was staring. Even the teacher! And after I sat down I could tell people were looking and laughing at me. Then when Ms. Ruby was done teaching and I was doing practice problems, my heart started beating and my skin was sweating and my hands were shaking and I just had to leave. And today I was so anxious that I just couldn't. So I skipped math.

> Therapist: Wow, I'm sorry this happened. It sounds like today your anxiety was high on that 1-to-10 scale we talked about. Where was it?

Summarizing integrates larger conversations into key concepts. It may simplify complex information, offer a new perspective, include action items, and also detail the next steps in therapy.

Accuracy, of course, is critical. An inaccurate paraphrase or summary may undermine confidence in the counseling process. Continuing with the example above:

> Client: Hmmm, I guess my anxiety was a 9 out of 10. I don't know if I can go back tomorrow, either, and we have a test review!
> Therapist: Let me know if I understand what happened to you correctly. Yesterday you tripped in the hallway. In class, after you thought people were staring and laughing at you, your anxiety got so high that you had to leave. The experience was so bad that today you avoided math class completely and worry you might not be able to go back. [Summary of events with an invitation for the client to correct the therapist if the summary is inaccurate]
> Client: Yep, that's it.
> Therapist: Sounds like that pattern of avoidance in social situations that we talked about last time. And it sounds like avoiding class in the short term is making the anxiety worse in the long run. [Reviews concept of avoidance; offers new perspective on worsening anxiety over time]
> Client: Huh. Yeah. I guess so. So, uh, what do we do? [Therapist can now summarize specific action steps.]

Reflection of Feelings

Reflection of feelings is an opportunity for the therapist to paraphrase the client's feelings. In addition, it is an opportunity to help clients build emotional insight and affix labels to their emotions. Therapists who do not listen carefully or accurately may misunderstand the valence of their client's feelings, resulting in the client feeling unheard or misunderstood. Here is a client statement followed by an effective response:

> Client: My new puppy got sick and died. This feeling is really bad. It makes my stomach hurt. I cried all day and don't feel good.
> Counselor: When you talk about your puppy dying, I hear the hurt in your voice. It sounds like you are feeling very sad. Is that right?

And this is what not to do:

> Counselor: When you talk about your puppy, it sounds like you think you did something bad. Are you feeling sick also?

THERAPEUTIC ALLIANCE

The therapeutic alliance, also called the working alliance, is "a cooperative working relationship between client and therapist, considered by many to be an essential aspect of successful therapy" (APA Dictionary of Psychology, n.d.). The concept is frequently credited to Edward Bordin (Bordin, 1979), though some authors think its roots may extend as far back as Freud's concept of transference (Horvath & Luborsky, 1993). In early influential research on the therapeutic alliance, Strupp and Hadley (1979) explored aspects of human relationships that could contribute to client success in psychotherapy, termed nonspecific factors. It is thought that the alliance is developed through these nonspecific factors, or interpersonal characteristics that encompass more than just the technical skills of counseling (Ackerman & Hilsenroth, 2003). Nonspecific factors include empathic responses, unconditional appreciation, respectful attention to differing opinions, need- and resource-oriented procedures, and stimulation of hope and reassurance (Bäuml et al., 2006). A strong therapeutic alliance could suggest a better client/therapist match than evaluating the match solely based on technical skills (Shirk & Saiz, 1992).

In a review of the role of nonspecific factors in CBT for depression, the largest amount of symptom improvement occurred before the formal treatment methods (or specific factors) were implemented (Ilardi & Craighead, 1994). Corroborating the research on this concept in their review of the history and literature on therapeutic alliance, Ardito and Rabellino (2011) also found that therapeutic alliance is a good predictor of counseling outcomes regardless of the specific counseling methods implemented. These findings highlight the importance and relevance of nonspecific factors in clinical treatment settings by suggesting that aspects of the therapist/client relationship can be healing independent of the therapy content. This information is useful for clinicians to consider when reflecting on their style and approach.

SUMMARY

In summary, students often enter counseling when distressed and sometimes without their input on the referral. Employing counseling micro skills in communication and purposefully striving to build therapeutic alliance can facilitate a more comfortable and productive experience. Counseling micro skills consist of five basic listening sequence components: client observation, attending, open/closed-ended questions, encouraging/ paraphrasing/summarizing, and reflection of feelings. Each technique is designed to enhance the communication and insight for both the counselor and student during sessions. These strategies provide dignity and respect to the client while also enhancing the building of trust.

CHAPTER DISCUSSION QUESTIONS

1. Compare and contrast FERPA and HIPAA provisions that may intersect within school practice.
2. What are the ethical guidelines for obtaining consent for counseling children and adolescents?
3. What are the ethical considerations in recordkeeping?
4. Discuss key factors that guide a practitioner's decision to provide group versus individual therapy.
5. What is the evidence for the effectiveness of including homework activities in counseling?
6. What are the core micro skills of counseling?
7. Describe factors that enhance therapeutic alliance.

REFERENCES

Ackerman, S. J., & Hilsenroth, M. J. (2003). A review of therapist characteristics and techniques positively impacting the therapeutic alliance. *Clinical Psychology Review*, *23*(1), 1–33. https://doi.org/10.1016/S0272-7358(02)00146-0

American Counseling Association. (2014). *ACA code of ethics: As approved by the ACA governing council*. Retrieved October 8, 2019, from https://www.counseling.org/docs

American Psychological Association. (2007). Record keeping guidelines. *American Psychologist*, *62*(9), 993–1004.

American Psychological Association. (2017). *Ethical principles of psychologists and code of conduct: Including 2010 and 2016 amendments*. Retrieved June 2, 2020, from https://www.apa.org/ethics/code/

APA Dictionary of Psychology. (n.d.) *Therapeutic alliance*. https://dictionary.apa.org/therapeutic-alliance

Ardito, R. B., & Rabellino, D. (2011). Therapeutic alliance and outcome of psychotherapy: Historical excursus, measurements, and prospects for research. *Frontiers in Psychology*, *2*, Article 270. https://doi.org/10.3389/fpsyg.2011.00270

Bäuml, J., Froböse, T., Kraemer, S., Rentrop, M., & Pitschel-Walz, G. (2006). Psychoeducation: A basic psychotherapeutic intervention for patients with schizophrenia and their families. *Schizophrenia Bulletin*, *32*(Suppl 1), S1–S9. https://doi.org/10.1093/schbul/sbl017

Bordin, E. S. (1979). The generalizability of the psychoanalytic concept of the working alliance. *Psychotherapy: Theory, Research and Practice*, *16*(3), 252–260. https://doi.org/10.1037/h0085885

Child Welfare Information Gateway. (2019). *Mandatory reporters of child abuse and neglect*. U.S. Department of Health and Human Services, Children's Bureau.

Coffman, C., & Barnett, J. E. (2015, October). *Informed consent with children and adolescents*. http://www.societyforpsychotherapy.org/informed-consent-with-children-and-adolescents

Daniels, T. (2010). A review of research on microcounseling: 1967–present. In A. Ivey, M. Ivey, & C. Zalaquett (Eds.), *Intentional interviewing and counseling: Your interactive resource* [CD-ROM]. Brooks/Cole.

Daniels, T., & Ivey, A. (2007). *Microcounseling: Making skills training work in a multicultural world*. Charles C. Thomas Pub. Ltd.

Edemekong, P. F., Annamaraju, P., & Haydel, M. J. (2020). *Health Insurance Portability and Accountability Act (HIPAA)*, StatPearls Publishing. Retrieved June 12, 2020, from https://www.ncbi.nlm.nih.gov/books/NBK500019/

Egan, G. (2007). *The skilled helper: A problem-management and opportunity-development approach to helping* (8th ed.). Brooks/Cole.

Eiraldi, R., Power, T. J., Schwartz, B. S., Keiffer, J. N., McCurdy, B. L., Mathen, M., & Jawad, A. F. (2016). Examining effectiveness of group cognitive-behavioral therapy for externalizing and internalizing disorders in urban schools. *Behavior Modification, 40*(4), 611–639. https://doi.org/10.1177/0145445516631093

Family Educational Rights and Privacy Act of 1974, 20 U.S.C. § 1232g (1974).

Health Insurance Portability and Accountability Act of 1996 (HIPAA) Pub. L. No. 104-191, 110 Stat. 1938 (1996).

Hill, C. E. (2004). *Dream work in therapy: Facilitating exploration, insight, and action*. American Psychological Association.

Horvath, A. O., & Luborsky, L. (1993). The role of the therapeutic alliance in psychotherapy. *Journal of Consultation and Clinical Psychology, 61*, 561–573. https://doi.org/10.1037/0022-006X.61.4.561

Ilardi, S. S., & Craighead, W. E. (1994). The role of nonspecific factors in cognitive behavioral therapy for depression. *Clinical Psychology Science and Practice, 1*(2), 138–155. https://doi.org/10.1111/j.1468-2850.1994.tb00016.x

Ivey, A. E., Ivey, M. B., & Zalaquett, C. P. (2017). *Intentional interviewing and counseling: Facilitating client development in a multicultural society* (9th ed.). Brooks/Cole.

Kazantzis, N., Deane, F. R., & Ronon, K. R. (2000). Meta-analysis of homework effects in cognitive and behavioral therapy: A replication and extension. *Clinical Psychology Science and Practice, 17*(2), 144–156.

Keles, S., & Idsoe, T. (2018). A meta-analysis of group cognitive behavioral therapy (CBT) interventions for adolescents with depression. *Journal of Adolescence, 18*(67), 129–139. doi:10.1016/j.adolescence.2018.05.011

Mausbach, B. T., Moore, R., Roesch, S., Cardenas, V., & Patterson, T. L. (2010). The relationship between homework compliance and therapy outcomes: An updated meta-analysis. *Cognitive Therapy and Research, 34*(5), 429–438. https://doi.org/10.1007/s10608-010-9297-z

Mitchell, R. W. (2007). *Documentation in counseling records: An overview of ethical, legal, and clinical issues* (3rd ed.). American Counseling Association.

National Association of School Psychologists. (2020). *Professional standards of the National Association of School Psychologists*. Author.

Santiago-Poventud, L., Corbett, N. L., Daunic, A. P., Aydin, B., Lane, H., & Smith, S. W. (2015). Developing social-emotional vocabulary to support self-regulation for young children at risk for emotional and behavioral problems. *International Journal of School and Cognitive Psychology, 2*(3), Article 143. https://doi.org/10.4172/2469-9837.1000143

Shirk, S. R., & Saiz, C. C. (1992). Clinical, empirical, and developmental perspectives on the therapeutic relationship in child psychotherapy. *Development and Psychopathology, 4*(4), 713–728.

Snyder, T. A., & Barnett, J. E. (2006). Informed consent and the psychotherapy process. *Psychotherapy Bulletin, 41*, 37–42.

Strupp, H. H., & Hadley, S. W. (1979). Specific vs. nonspecific factors in psychotherapy: A controlled study of outcome. *Archives of General Psychiatry, 36*(10), 1125–1136. https://doi.org/10.1001/archpsyc.1979.01780100095009

Truax, C. B., & Carkhuff, R. R. (1967). *Toward effective counseling and psychotherapy: Training and practice.* Aldine Publishing Company.

U.S. Department of Education. (2020). *Family Education Rights and Privacy Act (FERPA).* Retrieved May 1, 2020, from https://www2.ed.gov/policy/gen/guid/fpco/ferpa/index.html

U.S. Department of Health and Human Services. (2020). *Health information privacy.* Retrieved on April 3, 2020, from https://www.hhs.gov/hipaa/index.html

U.S. Department of Health and Human Services & U.S. Department of Education. (2008). *Joint guidance on the application of the Family Educational Rights and Privacy Act (FERPA) and the Health Insurance Portability and Accountability Act of 1996 (HIPAA) to student health records.* Retrieved May 1, 2020, from https://www.wrightslaw.com/info/ferpa.jointguide.doe.pdf

Zaboski, B. A., Joyce-Beaulieu, D., Kranzler, J. H., McNamara, J. P., Gayle, C., & MacInnes, J. (2019). Group exposure and response prevention for college students with social anxiety: A randomized clinical trial. *Journal of Clinical Psychology, 75*(9), 1489–1507. doi:10.1002/jclp.22792

Zhou, X., Zhang, Y., Furukawa, T. A., Cuijpers, P., Pu, J., Weisz, J. R., Yang, L., Hetrick, S. E., Del Giovane, C., Cohen, D., James, A. C., Yuan, S., Whittington, C., Jiang, X., Teng, T., Cipriani, A., & Xie, P. (2018). Different types and acceptability of psychotherapies for acute anxiety disorders in children and adolescents: A network meta-analysis. *JAMA Psychiatry, 76*(1), 41–50. doi:10.1001/jamapsychiatry.2018.3070

4

Culturally Responsive Mental Health Services

JANISE S. PARKER, DIANA JOYCE-BEAULIEU, AND
BRIAN A. ZABOSKI ■

Schools across the United States are becoming increasingly diverse. The National Center of Educational Statistics (NCES) projects a 6% decrease in students identifying as White by the year 2022, a 2% increase in students identifying as Black/African American, a 33% increase in students identifying as Hispanic, a 20% increase in students identifying as Asian/Pacific Islander, and a 44% increase in students identifying with two or more races (Hussar & Bailey, 2013). Although the NCES projects fewer than 5% of students identifying as American Indian/Alaska Native, these students, like other racial/ethnic minorities, are likely to have unique school and lived experiences that should be considered by school-based practitioners (e.g., substance abuse and disproportionate school discipline; Chen et al., 2012; Gregory et al., 2010).

In recognition of the growing diversity among K–12 students, researchers and educators continue to emphasize equitable treatment and support among culturally diverse learners (e.g., Darling-Hammond, 2010; Gregory et al., 2010). For example, school-based mental health services have garnered much attention in research and practice due to their promise as a viable means to reduce barriers to mental health care among students of color (Suldo et al., 2014). Compared to their White peers, students of color are less likely to access mental health support outside of the school setting due to structural and sociopolitical constraints, including poverty, lack of insurance, and the limited availability of behavioral health services in minority neighborhoods (Alegria et al., 2010; Thomas et al., 2011). School-based mental health services are presumed to address these constraints by offering accessible low-cost services for school-aged youth. Such services may include the implementation of social-emotional learning programs for all students or small group/individualized counseling (Macklem, 2011; National Association of School Psychologists [NASP], 2015).

Although evidence suggests that students of color may have equitable access to school mental health providers and support compared to their White peers (e.g., U.S. Department of Education, 2014), it is important to acknowledge that most school employees (including school mental health providers) are White/Non-Hispanic (e.g., Taie & Goldring, 2018; Walcott & Hyson, 2018). Consequently, school mental health providers may have remarkably different life experiences from the racial/ethnic minorities they serve. Such differences must not be overlooked, given that cultural mismatch may pose a major barrier to mental health care. For instance, racial/ethnic minorities may be less inclined to utilize mental health support when treatment providers do not take into consideration their lived experiences and cultural beliefs/values (e.g., Haboush, 2007; Hodge et al., 2009; Kouyoumdjian et al., 2003; Taylor et al., 2000).

In addition to diverse racial and ethnic experiences, researchers and practitioners have also recognized the varied experiences of LGBTQ+ youth (e.g., Kosciw et al., 2009) and religiously/spiritually diverse youth (Kim & Esquivel, 2011). In part, such attention has been influenced by the psychological distress and peer victimization experienced by youth who are in the minority on the basis of their sexual orientation, gender identity, or religion/spirituality (e.g., Atwal & Wang, 2019; Dupper et al., 2015; Goforth et al., 2017; Kosciw et al., 2009; Russell & Fish, 2016). Moreover, researchers now acknowledge that some students' cultural strengths—like religion/spirituality—have been overlooked for too long (Kim & Esquivel, 2011).

Considering that human diversity encompasses more than just race/ethnicity, practitioners should remember that cultural match is not limited to the shared (or divergent) racial/ethnic identities between themselves and the students they serve. To this end, school mental health providers must appreciate that one's racial/ethnic status alone does not guarantee a clinician's capacity to provide culturally responsive services. Evidence of such was demonstrated in the study conducted by Jones et al. (2016), wherein the researchers found that even clinicians of color struggled to provide culturally responsive support when serving clients from various cultural backgrounds, based on their age, disability status, and sexual orientation.

CULTURALLY RESPONSIVE THERAPY

Broadly defined, culturally responsive practice includes the purposeful use of targeted interventions that build on and align with individuals' cultural backgrounds, beliefs, and values (Jones, 2014). Culturally skilled counselors maintain cultural self-awareness, develop a cultural understanding of their clients, and provide individualized treatment in accordance with their clients' cultural needs (Sue et al., 1992). Within the context of cognitive behavioral therapy (CBT), this may include building on clients' strengths; validating their self-reported experiences of oppression; questioning the helpfulness (rather than the validity) of their thoughts or beliefs; and refraining from challenging their core beliefs (Hays, 2009).

Who Is the Client?

According to the *Professional Standards of the National Association of School Psychologists* (NASP, in press), the client is the "person with whom the school psychologist establishes a professional relationship for the purpose of providing school psychological services" (p. 52). In this regard, the student is typically identified as the client of school mental health services, though school psychologists may also support families, communities, and other school personnel. Because school psychologists are expected to provide culturally responsive support for the clients they serve, culturally adapted mental health services should align with the students' values, customs, and belief systems. Such consideration is especially critical when important aspects of their cultural identity are incongruent with their parents' values, customs, and beliefs. For example, immigrant youth may experience acculturative stress as they seek to navigate the tension between the development of their own identity and the familial pressures to maintain their cultural heritage (Goforth et al., 2016). Likewise, LGBTQ+ youth may experience interpersonal and intrapersonal difficulties when parents view the youth's sexual orientation and gender identity as incompatible with their religious/spiritual belief system (Duarté-Vélez et al., 2010; Yarhouse & Tan, 2005). By recognizing the student's unique cultural experiences, clinicians can create a safe space for the student to discuss and address culturally related issues in session.

Nevertheless, school-based mental health providers must also remember that because parents have the right to consent to school-based counseling, their perceptions should be acknowledged when considering the cultural responsiveness of the treatment plan. For example, in a study examining school psychologists' experiences with serving religiously/spiritually diverse students and families, one participant recounted a family's hesitance to utilize school-based mental health support for their child due to their desire to pray about the student's difficulties (Parker & Hanson, 2019). The school psychologist affirmed the family's cultural strength (praying as a coping mechanism) and recommended that the school *add* prayer to their intervention (vs. communicating that praying was ineffective). In turn, the family agreed to utilize the school-based mental health services provided for their child. Overall, school-based mental health providers should gain culturally relevant insight from all family members to aid case conceptualization and treatment planning.

Developmental Considerations

When providing culturally responsive services for school-aged youth, clinicians might consider adopting a developmental perspective to help youth reconcile the challenges of identity development (Nakkula & Toshalis, 2006). Several theories outline the process of identity development within the context of exploring and accepting one's cultural identity. Some of the presented stage-based theories recognize that individuals can fluctuate between stages or experience characteristics of "distinct" stages simultaneously. Finally, as many of the theories are based on general observations or group-level studies, they may not apply to all individuals; rather, they should be used as a guide for enriching case conceptualizations.

Gender

Bernal and Coolhart (2012) described the process of gender development among transgender and non-transgender youth in terms of Kohlberg's (1966) theory of gender consistency and Brill and Pepper's (2008) discussion of six developmental stages. According to Kohlberg's theory, children develop their gender identity in the preschool years, followed by an acknowledgment of gender stability (understanding they will grow up to be a woman or man) and gender consistency (accepting that they cannot change their gender). Bernal and Coolhart (2012) agree that transgender children also experience gender identity development during preschool but emphasized that Kohlberg's theory did not completely describe the unique developmental experiences of transgender youth. For example, they argue that transgender youth will also begin to recognize that their inner self does not match gender-related expectations as communicated by individuals in their environment (Bernal & Coolhart, 2012).

Due to the questionable applicability of Kohlberg's theory to transgender youth, Brill and Pepper (2008) highlighted six developmental stages uniquely experienced by this population. The first two stages occur between ages 2 and 4. During these stages the child will begin to classify males and females and express confusion about gender-variant adults. Next, children will likely gain awareness of anatomical gender differences and gender stereotypes/schemas (closer to ages 3 and 4). During this stage transgender children may express dissatisfaction or discomfort with their assigned gender. Between the ages of 4 and 6, transgender children may begin to believe they can grow up to be another gender. Thus, they may start rejecting expectations associated with their assigned gender. On the other hand, between the ages of 5 and 7, transgender children may acknowledge that one's gender is relatively stable based on societal expectations. This understanding may result in discomfort or behavioral/mental health problems if children are forced to limit their expression to their non-preferred gender. During the fifth stage, which occurs between the age of 9 and 12, gender identity becomes stronger with pubertal changes. Transgender youth may experience significant distress due to recognizing that changes in their bodies are inconsistent with their preferred gender. They also may continue to experience pressure to conform to their non-preferred gender, especially from peers. Finally, adolescents between the ages of 12 and 19 will feel like they are going through the wrong puberty, which may further perpetuate social and emotional concerns.

SEXUALITY

Researchers have published several frameworks on sexual identity development in LGBTQ+ individuals. With at least 16 stage theories included in the literature, Eliason and Schope (2007) highlighted some themes across the models. First, the process of homosexual identity development typically begins with the person feeling different in comparison to social norms. Second, individuals progress from low self-acceptance (accompanied by poor psychological adjustment) to a firm identity characterized by self-acceptance of one's sexual orientation. Third, LGBTQ+ individuals often feel a need to disclose their sexual orientation to others, where the "closeted" individual is viewed as less healthy than the open individual. Fourth, individuals from this community will feel a need to develop a sense of pride and cultural immersion, in which they are likely to surround themselves with other LGBTQ+ individuals. Last, individuals will feel a need to integrate their gender and sexual identities with other aspects of their personality.

FAITH

James Fowler's faith development theory is likely the best-known theory focused on faith development from childhood to adulthood (Fowler, 1981). Though Fowler defined faith more broadly than religiosity (e.g., his theory underscores how individuals begin to trust and rely on other people), the theory also includes special consideration of religious and spiritual development. During stage 1 (intuitive-projective faith), which generally occurs during the preschool age, children's faith may reflect fantasy-filled thoughts and behaviors rather than an organized set of ideas. For example, notions of God may be understood similarly to their comprehension of superheroes. Because faith is not yet identified as a cohesive set of tenets, adherence to religious customs is primarily encouraged by parents and other influential adults.

During stage 2 (mythic-literal faith), which typically occurs between ages 6 and 12, youth begin to think more logically and concretely. Stories and myths are interpreted in a more literal sense; thus, their faith is based on the stories told and rituals practiced. Perspective taking, defined as one's capacity to understand how others may think or feel about something, occurs later in this stage as children begin to understand that others may have different beliefs from them. During stage 3 (synthetic-conventional faith), which occurs between ages 13 and 18, adolescents begin to think more abstractly, with stories and rituals guiding their values and morals. Individuals at this stage also claim their faith as their own. Hence, adolescents may express a strong affinity to their religious/spiritual beliefs. According to Fowler's theory the last three stages (individuative-reflective faith, conjunctive faith, and universalizing faith) are likely to occur later in adulthood. People begin to question their own assumptions (and may leave their religious community), take more ownership of their faith, and engage in more self-reflection. Some individuals will open themselves to other faith perspectives and commit to contributing to the betterment of the world through faith-based practices.

Race

There are several models of racial/ethnic identity, such as those related to Chicano identity, Asian American identity, White identity, Black identity, and Indigenous American identity (Nakkula & Toshalis, 2006). Due to space limitations, we will limit our discussion to Cross's model of Black identity as it is one of the most popular theories in the literature. It describes how Blacks/African Americans obtain a psychologically healthy identity within the context of their interactions with White individuals (Cokley, 2002; Cross, 1995). Each stage in Cross's model describes behaviors, thoughts, and feelings Black individuals may experience in the process of developing a healthy cultural identity.

The first stage (pre-encounter) includes three distinct identity domains: (a) having a low salience for race but a strong orientation toward being an American, (b) internalizing negative stereotypes about being Black, or (c) holding extremely negative views about Black people, including themselves (self-hating). The second stage (encounter) occurs when one encounters discrimination or racism, causing a shift in their worldview and their identity. During the third stage (immersion-emersion), individuals will immerse themselves in intense Black involvement while rejecting White or Eurocentric views. Individuals may also experience anxiety about being or becoming "Black enough" given their newfound affinity for their racial identity. The fourth and fifth stages (internalization and internalization-commitment) reflect a period of pro-Black or Afrocentric orientation. Individuals integrate racial identity with other aspects of themselves and commit to demonstrating a concern for Black individuals as a collective group. They might also develop meaningful relationships with White individuals, if these individuals acknowledge and respect their self-identity.

Ethnicity

Phinney's (1989) model of adolescent ethnic identity is a well-established model for understanding ethnic development among adolescent students (Nakkula & Toshalis, 2006). In the first stage (unexamined ethnic identity), young people may either express little interest in their ethnic identity or adopt the positive ethnic attitudes expressed by parents or other adults. Regarding the latter, adolescents may show a preference for their ethnic group of affiliation, even if they have not given much thought to their presumed identity. In the second stage (ethnic identity search), adolescents may reject the values of the dominant culture to preserve the salience of their ethnicity. As such, adolescents may immerse themselves in their own culture by reading texts, speaking in their native language, attending cultural events, etc. When the identity search settles, adolescents will likely have a deeper appreciation of their ethnic identity and more confidence in it (achieved ethnic identity). They also will recognize cultural differences between their own group and the dominant group, including the lower status their group may have in society.

CHALLENGES RELATED TO MENTAL HEALTH

Because young children notice cultural-related differences across individuals, school counselors may need to help young children cope with social, emotional, and behavioral challenges emerging from their growing identities. Adolescents, however, will likely have more wherewithal to understand and communicate the interpersonal and intrapersonal implications of their cultural identity (Nakkula & Toshalis, 2006). They may also experience more psychological distress when their identity is not affirmed or supported by others or when it is viewed as incompatible with other aspects of their identity.

Identity-related psychological distress is well documented in professional scholarship. Research shows notable associations between (a) racially/ethnically diverse students' mental health and their experiences with racism, discrimination, and acculturative stress (Priest et al., 2013; Sirin et al., 2013) and (b) LGBTQ+ students' mental health and their experiences with discrimination, social isolation, and identity development/acceptance (Espelage et al., 2018; Kelleher, 2009; Russell & Fish, 2016). Religiously and spiritually diverse youth may experience psychological distress as well due to communicating an extreme fixation on salvation (Wagener & Mahoney, 2006) or attempting to navigate the tension between their religious/spiritual identity and their sexual orientation (Duarté-Vélez et al., 2010; Yarhouse & Tan, 2005). Furthermore, religious/spiritual minority youth may experience social isolation and religious-based bullying in school, which can impact their mental well-being (e.g., Dupper et al., 2015).

We recognize that other areas of human diversity are important to address when considering their interaction with students' psychological well-being: (a) age/generational influences, (b) disability status, (c) indigenous heritage, (d) national origin, and (e) socioeconomic status (Hays, 2009). However, due to space constraints, most of our discussion is focused on race/ethnicity, gender, sexuality, and religion/spirituality. For a compendium on child and adolescent developmental theories across these topics see Hupp and Jewel (2019).

MANAGING TREATMENT BARRIERS

Culturally diverse clients may be more receptive to maintaining the therapeutic relationship when the mental health provider acknowledges and values their lived experiences (Jones et al., 2016; Zigarelli et al., 2016). Drawing from Sue et al.'s (1992) work, we discuss how school-based mental health providers can provide empathic multicultural counseling that reflects a commitment to understanding clients' cultural identities. We explain these considerations within the context of (a) building cultural self-awareness, (b) developing a cultural understanding of the client, and (c) providing individualized treatment matched to the client's cultural needs.

Building Cultural Self-Awareness

Developing cultural self-awareness is foundational to culturally responsive practice, as one's own beliefs, values, and assumptions impact the therapeutic relationship. Learning about one's cultural identity includes an exploration of privilege, values, and beliefs (Miranda, 2014). For example, mental health providers should be willing to explore sociopolitical phenomena that impact their clients' lives (e.g., experiences with oppression; Hays, 2009; Hope & Chappelle, 2015). If clients sense discomfort among their counselors due to political correctness or if practitioners avoid emotionally charged topics, clients may be less willing to discuss thoughts/feelings related to race and culture (Zigarelli et al., 2016). Hence, school mental health providers are encouraged to confront their own discomfort to avoid invalidating or masking the student's lived experiences. If aspects of the therapist's cultural identity interfere with their capacity to provide culturally sensitive care, they should consider recusing themselves from the client–therapist relationship and make an appropriate referral to someone with the requisite expertise.

There are five steps to developing cultural self-awareness (Miranda, 2014). First, practitioners acknowledge personal prejudices and biases to identify faulty assumptions that may lead to inequitable treatment. The second step involves awareness that cultural standards, attitudes, and beliefs might be different than their own. The third step entails valuing the existence of cultural diversity. From there, one must be willing to reach out to the community to develop cultural knowledge about different groups. For example, cultural brokers are members of a select cultural group who can assist non-members to understand the group's cultural values, beliefs, and customs. Cultural brokers can help clinicians understand key differences between their own culture and that of the client while gaining useful information about the student's cultural group (Griffin & Farris, 2010; Zigarelli et al., 2016). The fifth step encourages developing a comfort level in novel situations that involve working with ethnic minority populations. Through developing self-awareness, school-based providers can strengthen their interactions with the students they serve by demonstrating respect for students' cultural backgrounds and responding effectively to their lived experiences.

Developing an Understanding of the Client

Before working with a diverse student, the school-based mental health provider might have gained some knowledge about the student's cultural group through formal coursework, immersion-related experiences, professional conferences/presentations, self-study, consultation with colleagues, or collaboration with individuals who understand the customs and values of the group. Information gained about a student's cultural group can build rapport; however, there are often more differences within groups than between groups (Miranda, 2014). Consequently, practitioners must avoid stereotyping or assuming that the client's experiences are synonymous with all members of the identified group. Because such differences are likely influenced by cultural intersectionality, it is important that school psychologists respond to various aspects of students' cultural identities when providing culturally responsive care (Zigarelli et al., 2016).

School personnel can use the ADDRESSING framework as a mnemonic to remember the range of cultural factors that influence a student's needs (Hays, 2009):

Age and generational influences
Developmental disabilities
Disabilities acquired later in life
Religion and spiritual orientation
Ethnic and racial identity
Socioeconomic status
Sexual orientation
Indigenous heritage
National origin
Gender

To inform treatment goals and to plan sessions that account for a student's cultural identity, practitioners can assess these factors as part of counseling preparation. Additionally, the Jones Intentional Multicultural Interview Schedule (JIMIS) can be used as a clinical interviewing tool to acquire this information. The JIMIS is a semistructured interview protocol that was developed to align with the ADDRESSING framework and to assist communication about cultural factors that may serve as sources of strength or stress (Jones, 2014; Zigarelli et al., 2016).

Providing Individualized Treatment

When serving diverse students, counseling support should maintain the core elements of the treatment approach (for example, CBT) while embedding and responding to aspects of the student's cultural identity within the intervention. Clinicians can accomplish this goal by utilizing culturally relevant material, building on students' strengths, and helping students cope with unique cultural challenges.

Utilize Culturally Relevant Material

School mental health providers can utilize examples from students' cultural backgrounds and life experiences to illustrate key ideas. For instance, Ginsburg and Drake (2002) implemented school-based group CBT to treat anxiety disorders among African American adolescents. The intervention included key CBT components such as psychoeducation about anxiety, relaxation exercises, cognitive restructuring, and gradual exposures to feared stimuli (see Chapters 5 through 7 for these techniques). Although the clinicians utilized a manual-based intervention, the program was culturally adapted. Specifically, some of the examples were modified to include experiences that the students were likely to encounter (e.g., neighborhood crime, violence, financial hardships). After 10 weekly 45- to 50-minute sessions, the adolescents in the CBT group reported slightly lower levels of overall anxiety ($d = 0.26$) and social anxiety ($d = 0.12$) compared to a control.

Similarly, Graves et al. (2017) implemented the Strong Start program for African American elementary students. Strong Start is a social-emotional learning curriculum that includes elements of CBT in the intervention manual: psychoeducation (e.g., teach students how to manage their anger), cognitive restructuring (e.g., teach students to challenge maladaptive thoughts), and social skills training (teach students basic communication and friendship-making skills). In the spirit of providing culturally responsive support, Graves et al. tailored the intervention to reflect the experiences of African American students. For example, when instructing students about friendship-making skills, the researchers utilized books with stories about African American characters in lieu of the recommended books that did not include such representation. They found large treatment effects for self-competence ($d = 1.38$) and self-regulation ($d = 0.99$) compared to a control group.

Build on Cultural Strengths

Students' cultural strengths can be directly integrated into their treatment plans. For example, one study examined the results of a culturally adapted version of Strong Teens for Latinx students: Jóvenes Fuertes (Castro-Olivo, 2014). The content includes lessons on ethnic pride (a cultural strength for Latinos) in addition to traditional CBT skills, like cognitive reframing and problem-solving skills, to cope with acculturative stress. When delivered in a school setting, the researchers found large intervention effects on social-emotional learning knowledge ($d = 1.27$) and social-emotional resiliency ($d = 0.44$) compared to a control group.

Religion and spirituality are a source of strength for many school-aged youth (Kim & Esquivel, 2011). Indeed, scholars propose that spiritual/religious perspectives can be integrated within evidence-based techniques. For example, Boynton (2014) described a mindfulness-based CBT program, the HEALTHY, for anxiety and depression among school-aged youth. In addition to traditional CBT, the HEALTHY includes spiritual material, such as encouraging youth to connect with a higher power. Similarly, Walker and Hathaway's (2013) book *Spiritual Interventions in Child and Adolescent Psychotherapy* recommends embedding several spiritual/religious strategies into traditional psychotherapy. For instance, the clinician can support students' use of prayer and use of sacred texts to develop positive thoughts. To investigate the effects of incorporating religious/spiritual strategies into psychotherapy, one meta-analysis synthesized results from 97 studies (Captari et al., 2018). When compared to a secular intervention, the researchers found no difference in psychological distress ($g = 0.13$); however, they found moderate effects on spiritual outcomes measures ($g = 0.34$) that were retained at least 1 month later ($g = 0.33$). These results indicate that including spiritual/religious perspectives in therapy may not only address psychological distress as well as secular interventions but also helps meet clients' spiritual/religious needs.

Help Students Cope with Culturally Related Challenges

Like teaching students how to cope with acculturative stress, culturally responsive treatment plans may consist of helping students manage interpersonal and intrapersonal challenges associated with their identity. As an example, transgender-affirmative CBT (TA-CBT) utilizes (a) psychoeducation to help the client understand the effects of anti-transgender attitudes and behaviors on their psychological well-being, (b) cognitive restructuring to increase positive thinking and challenge transphobic thoughts, (c) behavioral activation to encourage the client to participate in identity-affirming activities, and (d) social skills training to encourage social network building and to help the client respond to discrimination (Austin & Craig, 2015).

CASE EXAMPLES

Two case studies are presented here as examples of culturally-responsive CBT applications.

Audra

The first used CBT for a 15-year-old African American girl named Audra (Zigarelli et al., 2016). Audra worried about school, had trouble falling asleep, reported loneliness, wanted to run away, and believed life was unfair. She also experienced communication difficulties with her family and experienced frequent mood fluctuations. As such, Audra was referred to counseling to address her anxiousness, loneliness, and irritability.

In addition to a clinical interview, the therapist administered the Behavioral Assessment System for Children-Second Edition (BASC-2; Reynolds & Kamphaus, 2006) and the Reynolds Adolescent Depression Scale-Second Edition (RADS-2; Reynolds, 2002) to assess her current strengths and challenges. The assessment indicated that Audra's symptoms were consistent with persistent depressive disorder (formerly known as dysthymia) and generalized anxiety disorder. Thus, the clinician targeted symptoms associated with anxiety and depression. The clinician also applied the JIMIS at the beginning of treatment to understand Audra's cultural background and enrich the treatment plan.

The clinician found that Audra was distressed about (a) her family's socioeconomic status (her mother experienced financial hardships as a single parent), (b) her father's abandoning the family when she was younger, and (c) the challenges she faced as an African American adolescent (e.g., struggling to accept indications of her race/ethnicity, like her hair). The clinician helped Audra address these problems by (a) challenging maladaptive thoughts that interfered with her capacity to develop a positive racial/ethnic identity, (b) reaching out to her extended family members as a source of support (this represented a personal, cultural strength), and (c) working with her mother to identify ways to solve problems, improve communication, and express herself effectively. Follow-up data showed that her scores on the RADS-2 were in the normal (i.e., average) range. Furthermore, Audra showed a marginal increase in her self-rating of dysphoric mood and a decrease in her somatic complaints. Her mother's ratings on the BASC-2 showed a decline in her emotional symptoms.

Leonardo

The second case involved CBT for a 16-year-old Puerto Rican male (Duarté-Vélez et al., 2010). Leonardo's major concerns were anxiousness, depression, and attention/concentration difficulties. Leonardo and his mother completed behavioral rating scales (e.g., the Children's Depression Inventory; Kovacs, 1992) and face-to-face interviews at pretreatment, during treatment, at posttreatment, and in follow-up meetings. Pretreatment data indicated that Leonardo met criteria for major depressive disorder, unspecified anxiety disorder, and attention-deficit/hyperactivity disorder. Importantly, he experienced significant stress and peer rejection for his homosexual identity. He also felt a conflict between his sexual orientation, his ethnic identity, and his religious/spiritual beliefs. As a Latino, his culture endorsed strict gender roles regarding masculinity (a concept referred to as machismo), and he viewed his homosexuality as morally wrong due to his religious beliefs. Exacerbating his difficulties, his parents were unsupportive of his sexual orientation. These experiences caused Leonardo to develop dysfunctional attitudes about himself, including homophobic beliefs.

The clinician adapted the CBT protocol to reduce symptoms of depression while simultaneously addressing the cultural conflicts. For example, the clinician utilized psychoeducation to introduce different ideas about the expression of homosexuality and discuss negative social perceptions toward homosexuality. Furthermore, the clinician affirmed Leonardo's sexual orientation by acknowledging and congratulating him for discussing his sexual orientation during therapy and using the sessions to focus on "coming out" to his parents. The clinician also helped Leonardo address maladaptive thoughts about his sexual orientation and his interpersonal interactions. Finally, the clinician guided the decision-making process for "coming out" by assessing the pros and cons, planning the timing, and modeling assertive communication. The therapist facilitated a joint session with Leonardo's mother at the end of the intervention to improve her understanding about homosexuality and encourage mutual respect.

Over time, Leonardo became empowered and comfortable with himself. He confronted his greatest fear (talking to his father about his sexuality) and acknowledged that his parents may never accept him. Leonardo reported a notable decrease in depression symptomology from baseline to 1 year after treatment, and he improved his self-concept at the end of treatment. A structural clinical interview also showed that he no longer met criteria for major depressive disorder, though he continued to meet criteria for nonspecified anxiety and for attention-deficit/hyperactivity disorder.

SUMMARY

This chapter has reviewed national trends in race/ethnicity population data and offered a rationale for the need for culturally responsive mental health awareness to best serve the needs of diverse students. Developmental identity models have been reviewed in lieu of stages that youth make progress through in acquiring their own understanding of themselves and their culture. Two research case studies were included to illustrate specific strategies for implementation.

CHAPTER DISCUSSION QUESTIONS

1. Discuss three important considerations in providing culturally responsive therapy.
2. What strategies may be utilized to reduce treatment barriers?
3. How might therapists build on a client's cultural strengths?
4. Discuss developmental considerations you would consider in planning counseling.
5. Discuss the standards and ethical guidelines related to determining who is the client.
6. What are some strategies to individualize culturally responsive therapy?
7. Discuss the five steps to developing self-awareness.

REFERENCES

Alegria, M., Vallas, M., & Pumariega, A. J. (2010). Racial and ethnic disparities in pediatric mental health. *Child and Adolescent Psychiatric Clinics, 19,* 759–774. https://doi.org/10.1016/j.chc.2010.07.001Atwal, K., & Wang, C. (2019). Religious head covering, being perceived as foreigners, victimization, and adjustment among Sikh American adolescents. *School Psychology, 34,* 233–243. https://doi.org/10.1037/spq0000301

Austin, A., & Craig, S. L. (2015). Transgender affirmative cognitive behavioral therapy: Clinical considerations and applications. *Professional Psychology: Research and Practice, 46*(1), 21–29. https://doi.org/10.1037/a0038642

Bernal, A. T., & Coolhart, D. (2012). Treatment and ethical considerations with transgender children and youth in family therapy. *Journal of Family Psychotherapy, 23*(4), 287–303. https://doi.org/10.1080/08975353.2012.735594

Boynton, H. M. (2014). The healthy group: A mind–body–spirit approach for treating anxiety and depression in youth. *Journal of Religion & Spirituality in Social Work: Social Thought, 33*(3–4), 236–253. https://doi.org/10.1080/15426432.2014.930629

Brill, S., & Pepper, R. (2008). *The transgender child: A handbook for families and professionals.* Cleis Press Inc.

Captari, L. E., Hook, J. N., Hoyt, W., Davis, D. E., McElroy-Heltzel, S. E., & Worthington Jr., E. L. (2018). Integrating clients' religion and spirituality within psychotherapy: A comprehensive meta-analysis. *Journal of Clinical Psychology, 74*(11), 1938–1951. https://doi.org/10.1002/jclp.22681

Castro-Olivo, S. M. (2014). Promoting social-emotional learning in adolescent Latino ELLs: A study of the culturally adapted Strong Teens program. *School Psychology Quarterly, 29*(4), 567–577. https://doi.org/10.1037/spq0000055

Chen, H. J., Balan, S., & Price, R. K. (2012). Association of contextual factors with drug use and binge drinking among White, Native American, and Mixed-Race adolescents in the general population. *Journal of Youth and Adolescence, 41*(11), 1426–1441. https://doi.org/10.1007/s10964-012-9789-0

Cokley, K. O. (2002). Testing Cross's revised racial identity model: An examination of the relationship between racial identity and internalized racialism. *Journal of Counseling Psychology, 49*(4), 476–483. https://doi.org/10.1037/0022-0167.49.4.476

Cross, W. E., Jr. (1995). The psychology of nigrescence: Revising the Cross model. In J. G. Ponterotto, J. M. Casas, L. A. Suzuki, & C. M. Alexander (Eds.), *Handbook of multicultural counseling* (pp. 93–122). Sage Publications, Inc.

Darling-Hammond, L. (2010). *The flat world and education: How America's commitment to equity will determine our future*. Teachers College Press.

Duarté-Vélez, Y., Bernal, G., & Bonilla, K. (2010). Culturally adapted cognitive-behavior therapy: Integrating sexual, spiritual, and family identities in an evidence-based treatment of a depressed Latino adolescent. *Journal of Clinical Psychology, 66*(8), 895–906. https://doi.org/10.1002/jclp.20710

Dupper, D. R., Forrest-Bank, S., & Lowry-Carusillo, A. (2015). Experiences of religious minorities in public school settings: Findings from focus groups involving Muslim, Jewish, Catholic, and Unitarian Universalist youths. *Children and Schools, 37*(1), 37–45. https://doi.org/10.1093/cs/cdu029

Eliason, M. J., & Schope, R. (2007). Shifting sands or solid foundation? Lesbian, gay, bisexual, and transgender identity formation. In I. H. Meyer, & M. E. Northridge (Eds.), *The health of sexual minorities: Public health perspectives on lesbian, gay, bisexual, and transgender populations* (pp. 3–26). Springer Science + Business Media, LLC. https://doi.org/10.1007/978-0-387-31334-4_1

Espelage, D. L., Merrin, G. J., & Hatchel, T. (2018). Peer victimization and dating violence among LGBTQ youth: The impact of school violence and crime on mental health outcomes. *Youth Violence and Juvenile Justice, 16*(2), 156–173. https://doi.org/10.1177/1541204016680408

Fowler, J. W. (1981). *Stages of faith: The psychology of human development and the quest for meaning*. HarperCollins.

Ginsburg, G. S., & Drake, K. L. (2002). School-based treatment for anxious African-American adolescents: A controlled pilot study. *Journal of the American Academy of Child & Adolescent Psychiatry, 41*(7), 768–775. https://doi.org/10.1097/00004583-200207000-00007

Goforth, A. N., Nichols, L. M., Stanick, C. F., Shindorf, Z. R., & Holter, O. (2017). School-based considerations for supporting Arab American youths' mental health. *Contemporary School Psychology, 21*(3), 191–200. https://doi.org/10.1007/s40688-016-0117-7

Goforth, A. N., Pham, A. V., Chun, H., Castro-Olivo, S. M., & Yosai, E. R. (2016). Association of acculturative stress, Islamic practices, and internalizing symptoms among Arab American adolescents. *School Psychology Quarterly, 31*(2), 198–212. https://doi.org/10.1037/spq0000135

Graves Jr., S. L., Herndon-Sobalvarro, A., Nichols, K., Aston, C., Ryan, A., Blefari, A., Schutte, K., Schachner, A., Vicoria, L., & Prier, D. (2017). Examining the effectiveness of a culturally adapted social-emotional intervention for African American males in an urban setting. *School Psychology Quarterly, 32*(1), 62–74. https://doi.org/10.1037/spq0000145

Gregory, A., Skiba, R. J., & Noguera, P. A. (2010). The achievement gap and the discipline gap: Two sides of the same coin? *Educational Researcher, 39*(1), 59–68. https://doi.org/10.3102/0013189X09357621

Griffin, D., & Farris, A. (2010). School counselors and collaboration: Finding resources through community asset mapping. *Professional School Counseling, 13*(5), 248–256. https://doi.org/10.1177/2156759X1001300501

Haboush, K. L. (2007). Working with Arab American families: Culturally competent practice for school psychologists. *Psychology in the Schools, 44*(2), 183–198. https://doi.org/10.1002/pits.20215

Hays, P. A. (2009). Integrating evidence-based practice, cognitive–behavior therapy, and multicultural therapy: Ten steps for culturally competent practice. *Professional Psychology: Research and Practice, 40*(4), 354–360. https://doi.org/10.1037/a0016250

Hodge, D. R., Limb, G. E., & Cross, T. L. (2009). Moving from colonization toward balance and harmony: A Native American perspective on wellness. *Social Work, 54*(3), 211–219. https://www.jstor.org/stable/23719497

Hope, D. A., & Chappell, C. L. (2015). Extending training in multicultural competencies to include individuals identifying as lesbian, gay, and bisexual: Key choice points for clinical psychology training programs. *Clinical Psychology: Science and Practice, 22*(2), 105–118. https://doi.org/10.1111/cpsp.12099

Hupp, S., & Jewel, J. D. (2019). *The encyclopedia of child and adolescent development.* John Wiley & Sons. doi:10.1002/9781119171492

Hussar, W. J., & Bailey, T. M. (2013). *Projections of education statistics to 2022* (NCES 2014-051). U.S. Department of Education, National Center for Education Statistics. https://nces.ed.gov/pubs2014/2014051.pdf

Jones, J. (2014). Best practices in providing culturally responsive interventions. In P. L. Harrison & A. Thomas (Eds.), *Best practices in school psychology: Foundations* (pp. 49–60). National Association of School Psychologists.

Jones, J. M., Kawena Begay, K., Nakagawa, Y., Cevasco, M., & Sit, J. (2016). Multicultural counseling competence training: Adding value with multicultural consultation. *Journal of Educational and Psychological Consultation, 26*(3), 241–265. https://doi.org/10.1080/10474412.2015.1012671

Kelleher, C. (2009). Minority stress and health: Implications for lesbian, gay, bisexual, transgender, and questioning (LGBTQ) young people. *Counselling Psychology Quarterly, 22*(4), 373–379. https://doi.org/10.1080/09515070903334995

Kim, S., & Esquivel, G. B. (2011). Adolescent spirituality and resilience: Theory, research, and educational practices. *Psychology in the Schools, 48*(7), 755–765. https://doi.org/10.1002/pits.20582

Kohlberg, L. (1966). A cognitive-developmental analysis of children's sex-role concepts and attitudes. In E. E. Maccoby (Ed.), *The development of sex differences* (pp. 82–173). Stanford University Press.

Kosciw, J. G., Greytak, E. A., & Diaz, E. M. (2009). Who, what, where, when, and why: Demographic and ecological factors contributing to hostile school climate for lesbian, gay, bisexual, and transgender youth. *Journal of Youth and Adolescence*, 38(7), 976–988. https://doi.org/10.1007/s10964-009-9412-1

Kouyoumdjian, H., Zamboanga, B. L., & Hansen, D. J. (2003). Barriers to community mental health services for Latinos: Treatment considerations. *Clinical Psychology: Science and Practice*, 10(4), 394–422. https://doi.org/10.1093/clipsy/bpg041

Kovacs, M. (1992). *Children's Depression Inventory manual*. Multi-Health Systems, Inc.

Macklem, G. L. (2011). Evidence-based tier 1, tier 2, and tier 2 mental health interventions in schools. In *Evidence-based school mental health services: Affect education, emotion regulation training, and cognitive behavioral therapy* (pp. 19–37). Springer Science and Business Media.

Miranda, A. H. (2014). Best practices in increasing cross-cultural competency. In P. L. Harrison & A. Thomas (Eds.), *Best practices in school psychology: Foundations* (pp. 9–20). National Association of School Psychologists.

Nakkula, M. J., & Toshalis, E. (2006). *Understanding youth: Adolescent development for educators*. Harvard Education Press.

National Association of School Psychologists. (2015). *School psychologists: Qualified health professionals providing child and adolescent mental and behavioral health services*. Author.

National Association of School Psychologists. (in press). *Professional Standards of the National Association of School Psychologists*. Author.

Parker, J. S., & Hanson, P. (2019). School stakeholders do not "just leave their religious beliefs at home": An exploratory study of school psychologists' professional experiences. *International Journal of School & Educational Psychology*, 1–13. https://doi.org/10.1080/21683603.2019.1666441

Phinney, J. S. (1989). Stages of ethnic identify development in minority group adolescents. *Journal of Early Adolescence*, 9(1–2), 34–49. https://doi.org/10.1177/0272431689091004

Priest, N., Paradies, Y., Trenerry, B., Truong, M., Karlsen, S., & Kelly, Y. (2013). A systematic review of studies examining the relationship between reported racism and health and wellbeing for children and young people. *Social Science & Medicine*, 95, 115–127. https://doi.org/10.1016/j.socscimed.2012.11.031

Reynolds, C. R., & Kamphaus, R. W. (2006). *BASC-2: Behavior Assessment System for Children, Second Edition*. Pearson Education.

Reynolds, W. M. (2002). *Reynolds Adolescent Depression Scale: Professional manual* (2nd ed.). Psychological Assessment Resources.

Russell, S. T., & Fish, J. N. (2016). Mental health in lesbian, gay, bisexual, and transgender (LGBT) youth. *Annual Review of Clinical Psychology*, 12, 465–487. https://doi.org/10.1146/annurev-clinpsy-021815-093153

Sirin, S. R., Ryce, P., Gupta, T., & Rogers-Sirin, L. (2013). The role of acculturative stress on mental health symptoms for immigrant adolescents: A longitudinal investigation. *Developmental Psychology*, 49(4), 736–748. https://doi.org/10.1037/a0028398

Sue, D. W., Arredondo, P., & McDavis, R. J. (1992). Multicultural counseling competencies and standards: A call to the profession. *Journal of Multicultural Counseling and Development*, 20(2), 64–88. https://doi.org/10.1002/j.1556-6676.1992.tb01642.x

Suldo, S. M., Gormley, M. J., DuPaul, G. J., & Anderson-Butcher, D. (2014). The impact of school mental health on student and school-level academic outcomes: Current status of the research and future directions. *School Mental Health, 6*, 84–98. https://doi.org/10.1007/s12310-013-9116-2

Taie, S., & Goldring, R. (2018). *Characteristics of public elementary and secondary school teachers in the United States: Results from the 2015–16 National Teacher and Principal Survey First Look* (NCES 2017-072rev). U.S. Department of Education, National Center for Education Statistics. https://nces.ed.gov/pubs2017/2017070.pdf

Taylor, R. J., Ellison, C. G., Chatters, L. M., Levin, J. S., & Lincoln, K. D. (2000). Mental health services in faith communities: The role of clergy in Black churches. *Social Work, 45*(1), 73–87.

Thomas, J. F., Temple, J. R., Perez, N., & Rupp, R. (2011). Ethnic and gender disparities in needed adolescent mental health care. *Journal of Health Care for the Poor and Underserved, 22*, 101–110. https://doi.org/10.1353/hpu.2011.0029

U.S. Department of Education. (2014). *Mental health staff in public schools, by school racial and ethnic composition.* https://nces.ed.gov/pubs2019/2019020.pdf

Wagener, L. M., & Mahoney, H. N. (2006). Spiritual and religious pathology in childhood and adolescence. In E. C. Roehlkepartain, P. E. King, L. M. Wagener, & P. L. Benson (Eds.), *The handbook of spiritual development in childhood and adolescence* (pp. 137–149). SAGE Publications, Inc.

Walcott, C. M., & Hyson, D. (2018). *Results from the NASP 2015 membership survey, part one: Demographics and employment conditions.* National Association of School Psychologists.

Walker, D. F., & Hathaway, W. L. (2013). *Spiritual interventions in child and adolescent psychotherapy.* American Psychological Association.

Yarhouse, M. A., & Tan, E. S. N. (2005). Addressing religious conflicts in adolescents who experience sexual identity confusion. *Professional Psychology: Research and Practice, 36*, 530–536. https://doi.org/10.1037/0735-7028.36.5.530

Zigarelli, J. C., Jones, J. M., Palomino, C. I., & Kawamura, R. (2016). Culturally responsive cognitive behavioral therapy: Making the case for integrating cultural factors in evidence-based treatment. *Clinical Case Studies, 15*(6), 427–442. https://doi.org/10.1177/1534650116664984

5

Psychoeducation, Relaxation Training, and Mindfulness

ANNA SCHRACK, EMMA ROMAKER, DIANA JOYCE-BEAULIEU, AND BRIAN A. ZABOSKI ■

Within the MTSS model of counseling supports, the greatest percentage of students served will have Tier 2 needs at a mild to moderate level. This chapter will offer foundational counseling components that may be applied as initial approaches for these needs. More intense and complex needs will require techniques reviewed in Chapters 6 and 7 (e.g., cognitive restructuring, behavioral activation, or exposure/response prevention).

PSYCHOEDUCATION

Psychoeducation is the process of sharing accurate information with clients and their support systems, usually in an organized and methodical manner that describes an intervention plan for problem behaviors or psychiatric illnesses. Goals include dispelling myths and misinformation about mental health, teaching clients the underlying or maintaining mechanisms and trajectory of mental health symptoms, exploring individualized treatment options, having candid discussions of medication effects, and fostering empowerment. Through this understanding, practitioners seek to increase the likelihood of intervention adherence, help clients provide more informed consent for services, and develop a common language for problems and solutions. In addition to providing information and motivation, psychoeducation may also help clients develop metacognition, or self-awareness of their own functioning and needs (Ekhtiari et al., 2017).

One of the key premises of psychoeducation suggests when that patients and families have acquired competency in understanding mental health struggles, they can better support, cope, and ameliorate symptoms (Bäuml et al., 2006). The inclusion of psychoeducation may be particularly important when mental health needs are severe, pervasive, and chronic and represent a lifetime struggle. For example, the article by Ekhtiari et al. (2017) discusses applications for mental health symptoms that often accompany low personal insight (alcohol or substance addiction). For these individuals and their families, therapists should provide comprehensive psychoeducation, frequently review information, monitor treatment engagement, and measure changes in insight.

Although not recommended as a standalone treatment modality, evidence suggests that augmenting interventions with psychoeducation confers several benefits. In a randomized trial of psychoeducation programming across multiple treatment centers for patients with schizophrenia and their families, researchers found positive short- and long-term results. At 2 years following program completion, patients with schizophrenia who were readmitted to the hospital dropped from 58% to 41%, and for those hospitalized, the length of stay fell from 78 days to 39 days (Bäuml et al., 2006). In a study on providing psychoeducation to parents and their 7- to 12-year-old children who were scheduled for surgery, researchers measured parent and child anxiety at three time points: preoperatively (before the intervention), on the day of surgery just before the operation (after the intervention), and on the day of surgery after the operation (Cheung et al., 2007). Both the matched control and experimental groups were provided the routine verbal explanation of the surgery process. However, those in the experimental group were also introduced to the surgical area and attire, were allowed to touch medical equipment (e.g., blood pressure cuff, anesthesia mask), and were given more detailed information on what to expect. The study found that the anxiety of both the parents and children who received psychoeducation was significantly lower before and after the surgery compared to matched controls.

Further establishing the utility of psychoeducation, a separate study investigated 652 children and adolescents with separated or divorced parents. The curriculum focused on eight key points to help children understand divorce: anger, substance abuse, feeling responsible for parents, pulled between parents, neglect, and verbal, physical, and sexual abuse. Eight questionnaires regarding these topics were administered before and after the intervention. The significant difference in scores indicated that students increased their understanding of changing family dynamics and common experiences that can stem from divorce (Slavkin, 2000).

We recommend delivering school-based psychoeducation in three phases: knowledge building, coping/compensating mechanisms, and empowerment (Figure 5.1; Joyce-Beaulieu, 2020).

Knowledge Building

In the first phase, an initial knowledge-building step for a student struggling with attention-deficit/hyperactivity disorder (ADHD) would include explaining the DSM-5 symptoms and what those symptoms might look like in daily life (e.g.,

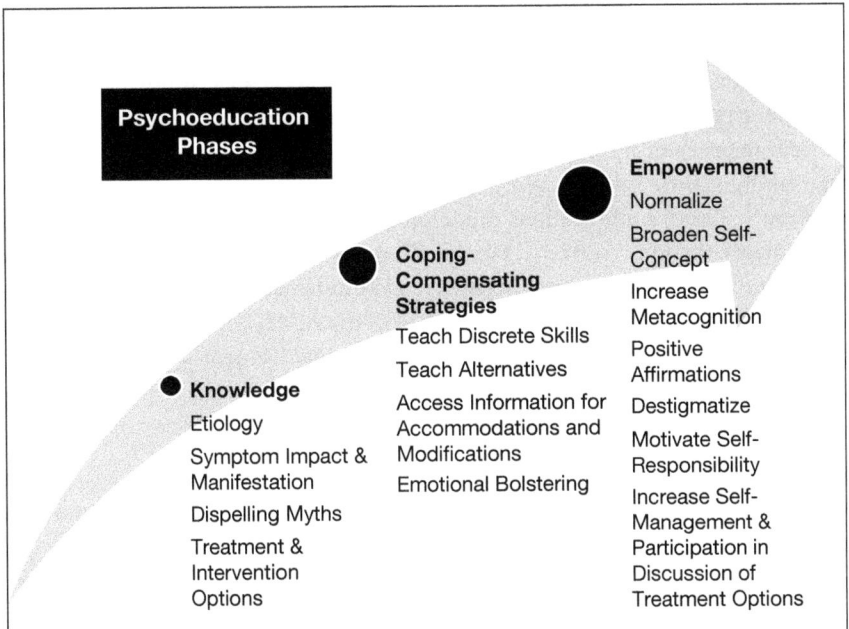

Figure 5.1 Psychoeducation Phases
(Joyce-Beaulieu, 2020)

forgetting homework, getting easily distracted, blurting impulsively instead of waiting one's turn).

Coping/Compensating Mechanisms

Second, coping/compensating mechanisms emphasize skills that help the student manage the symptoms (e.g., impulse control strategies for blurting, organizational skills for managing assignments, alternatives for movement/fidgeting, strategies for limiting extraneous stimuli, knowledge on accommodations and modifications). In this stage, emotional bolstering is also important, like acknowledging a student's extra efforts and achievements. This encouragement can take the form of praise, recognition, or incentives for completing personal goals. Students also may find it beneficial to join support groups to build insight and positive social interactions.

Empowerment

Third, empowerment includes normalizing and destigmatizing problems while identifying successful role models. By explaining the prevalence of ADHD and the fact that many students of all ages have ADHD, therapists can help normalize it. Practitioners can start to destigmatize ADHD by describing it as a neurological problem that is not a student's fault. Additionally, identifying successful individuals who have ADHD and achieve ambitious goals can normalize it and mitigate stigmatization. Moreover, empowerment involves teaching students to view themselves holistically by embracing their strengths and talents rather than limiting their self-concept (e.g., "I'm just a kid with a mental or physical problem"). Positive affirmations are another way of building self-concept (e.g., "I am bigger than my ADHD," "I am in charge of my ADHD," "ADHD is not the sum of me"). In this case, empowerment can be enhanced by encouraging ownership of one's symptoms ("I'm taking control of my ADHD"). For adolescents, empowerment and ownership can also mean more involvement with their medical providers and treatment decisions.

MOTIVATIONAL INTERVIEWING (MI)

MI is all about change. It acknowledges that change is an uphill battle for many people, filled with obstacles that vary from person to person. MI owes its popularity to William Miller, who shifted the widely held perspective in addiction treatment away from blaming clients for lacking motivation (Rollnick & Allison, 2004). The ideology behind MI was outlined in Miller's work on implementing this interviewing style with problem drinkers (Miller, 1983). Subsequently, MI became a mainstream treatment approach for alcoholism. In 1991, Miller and Rollnick revised the technique, and it was later adapted for application with client groups aside from those with addiction/alcohol problems (Miller & Rollnick, 1991). Some classic examples of alternative applications include cravings when trying to stop smoking, hunger pains when losing weight, or putting off doing household chores due to laziness. MI excels at addressing these difficulties and the ambivalence that accompanies change. Miller and Rollnick (2013) defined MI as:

> a collaborative, goal-oriented style of communication with particular attention to the language of change. It is designed to strengthen personal motivation for and commitment to a specific goal by eliciting and exploring the person's own reasons for change within an atmosphere of acceptance and compassion. (p. 43)

The "collaborative" component of the definition highlights the client–therapist dyad as a team, while "goal-oriented" emphasizes the goals that the client would like to focus on. Therapists attend to the language of change, which is nondirective and nonconfrontational. It does not force change to happen ("You have to quit smoking, or your health is at risk!") but rather cultivates a readiness for change ("If you were to stop smoking, is there any benefit to you?"). In MI, the client sets the goals while the therapist elicits and explores reasons for change. Through this perspective, the client is viewed as having the ability to change all along, and the therapist is just there to evoke it.

Throughout the process, the therapist creates an atmosphere of acceptance that allows clients to speak openly, conveying that they have worth and are in control of their life. This also allows the therapist to understand the client's perspective and to see the world as the client does. An atmosphere of compassion shows clients, through empathy and understanding, that the therapist has their best interests at heart. The core component of MI is that clients set the goals and make the changes, with the therapist helping them to understand their situation as it relates to their goals and what is needed to accomplish them.

Through strengthening a client's motivation for change, practitioners help resolve ambivalence, or a kind of hesitance, about change. This can be fostered through reflective listening, eliciting change talk, and a "change ruler."

Reflective Listening

Reflective listening (sometimes also known as paraphrasing—see Chapter 3) involves attending to the client and then checking one's understanding through phrasing a reflection of what was heard as a statement instead of a question. For example:

> Client: I guess I want to study more for the SAT, but I also really like to play video games.
> Therapist: What I'm hearing is that you want to study more, but a temptation to play video games can hold that back.

In this response, the therapist does not direct the client to any particular solution. Rather, the therapist paraphrases the problem and highlights the conflict between the client's desire to play video games and do well on the SAT.

Eliciting Change Talk

Eliciting change talk involves asking questions and phrasing statements so that the client uses language that indicates movement toward a goal. Continuing the previous example:

> Client: Yes! It's so frustrating! I hate feeling stuck.
> Therapist: Ahh, yes, I think most people can relate to that. It sounds like for you, progress might mean somehow resolving the tension between these two interests.
> Client: Eh, yeah, I guess it would be nice to move forward.

Note here that the therapist seized this opportunity to elicit change talk by mentioning "progress." Although the client may not yet be sold on this idea, therapists using MI encourage clients to grow accustomed to using the language of change.

Change Ruler

Another method of resolving ambivalence, a change ruler, involves asking clients to identify how ready, willing, and able they are to change. Note that these three qualities can be rated quite differently! Continuing the same example:

> Therapist: Are you ready for that?
> Client: I'm not sure.
> Therapist: Well, let's put it on one of our scales. How ready are you from 1 to 10?
> Client: Maybe a 4. I feel kinda torn.
> Therapist: How willing are you to give it a try?
> Client: Oh, I'd say about a 7. I want to try, I really do. I just don't know how ready I am.
> Therapist: On our 1-to-10 scale, how able are you to work on this right now?
> Client: Well, I'm definitely able. I feel like I'm the one holding myself back.

Although the client seems willing and able to change, there is still some ambivalence about readiness to change. Thus, by using the change ruler, the therapist gains information to explore during the rest of the session.

While MI was originally designed for use with individuals struggling with substance abuse, meta-analyses have also indicated its effectiveness with other conditions and settings. For example, when reviewing the efficacy of MI for health behavior outcomes in primary care settings, 9 out of the 12 studies displayed higher efficacy for MI than for the control conditions/standard procedures (VanBuskirk & Wetherell, 2014). Additionally, MI has been used as a pretreatment technique for people seeking treatment for mental health problems and those not seeking treatment. In one meta-analysis, for individuals who were not seeking treatment, a 15-minute MI intervention by phone quintupled their treatment attendance compared to treatment seekers (Lawrence et al., 2017). Thus, MI may work best for students who are ambivalent about seeking help.

Some research on MI has been mixed. For example, to evaluate the efficacy of empirically supported interventions for anxiety and depression in primary care, a systematic review and meta-analysis was conducted (Zhang et al., 2019). The overall treatment effect of MI across six studies was small ($d = 0.28$), though the results were not significant. A separate meta-analysis examining MI for children and adolescents also found a small effect across 37 studies ($g = 0.28$; Gayes & Steele, 2014). However, the authors note that the studies in the meta-analysis were heterogenous (a meta-analytic term for "different"), indicating that the effect size may be attenuated by factors other than the intervention. For instance, they found that community health workers (i.e., do not have a terminal degree) demonstrated the largest effects ($g = 0.49$), professional interventiontists (e.g., nurses) demonstrated similar effect sizes ($g = 0.36$) whereas master's- or doctoral-level interventionists had the smallest effects ($g = 0.24$). Similarly, MI with both parents and children present yielded larger effects than either party alone ($g = 0.59$). Despite these research challenges, MI shows promise for children and adolescents, especially when incorporated with the family and when there is high ambivalence for change.

RELAXATION TRAINING

When individuals experience fear or stress, sensory stimuli are sent to the part of the brain that processes emotion (amygdala), which then sends distress notices to the hypothalamus and subsequently activates the adrenal glands to release epinephrine (Arnsten, 1998; Harvard Health Publishing, 2020). This creates an almost instantaneous release of glucose and stored fat that allows the individual to react swiftly and with a high level of alertness. When the threat passes, the body can gradually relax. But if the fear or stress is sustained, the hypothalamus will activate additional hormone and cortisol release to maintain high-alert status. Regardless of whether the threat is misperceived or realistic, the body cannot maintain repeated and prolonged high-alert status without negative effects (Maughan & Cicchetti, 2003; Sherin & Nemeroff, 2011). Too much blood sugar (glucose) release and increased appetite can cause weight gain and obesity. Maintaining an accelerated heart rate can lead to high blood pressure, and some studies have found that chronic stress results in changes in the brain associated with addiction, depression, and anxiety (Harvard Health Publishing, 2020; Kessler et al., 2020; Sinha, 2008).

High levels of chronic stress, especially related to maltreatment or trauma, can impair emotion regulation, cognition, affective functioning, and the neuroimmune system in children and adolescents (Brenhouse et al., 2018; Maughan & Cicchetti, 2003; Pechtel & Pizzagalli, 2011). In a study of 189 children aged 4 to 6 years, 80% of children with a history of maltreatment exhibited disruptive emotional regulation compared to 37% of children without such a history (Maughan & Cicchetti, 2003). In a review of longitudinal neurobiological studies on brain development, significant early life stress was also associated with deficits in overall cognitive, executive, memory, reward processing, social/affective stimuli awareness, and emotional regulation functions (Pechtel & Pizzagalli, 2011). These deficits persisted for years after the adversity had ceased. Brenhouse et al. (2018) noted that children with significant early life maltreatment and trauma experienced dysfunctional immune development due to sustained, stress-related inflammation. Long-term consequences included over-reactive immune responses to stress years later. The failure to recover cognitive and affective functioning following a stressor could increase the likelihood of developing anxiety and mood disorders.

Relaxation training helps clients manage stressors by teaching them activities designed to reduce hypertensive physiological responses (perspiration, heart rate, blood pressure, or muscle tension) and decrease feelings of anxiety, stress, fear, or pain (Norelli et al., 2020). Through relaxation training, students also learn that stress, anxiousness, and fear are inescapable parts of the human experience and can even be beneficial. For example, a person who enjoys roller coasters may enjoy the stress response resulting from the ride, while someone with a fear of heights may not. A second example might be a student motivated to engage in additional practice prior to a basketball game given their anxiousness about performance. Most likely this extra practice will enhance their performance. This conundrum emphasizes that "bad stress" is situational and specific to each person and that short-term doses of stress can be productive, adaptive, and enjoyable (Thiel & Dretsch, 2011).

Relaxation exercises can target subjectively reported psychological feelings or observable physical responses and are utilized in psychology and the broader healthcare community (Norelli et al., 2020). The same techniques can be used to address physical and psychological needs simultaneously. Relaxation training has been adapted and utilized with children in school settings and has the potential to teach students methods and techniques to alleviate physiological stress responses (Lohaus et al., 2010; Zaichkowsky & Zaichkowsky, 1983). Additional benefits for relaxation training include improved quality of sleep, improved digestion, reduced fatigue, and lowered anger and frustration (Deffenbacher & Stark, 1992; Harvard Health Publishing, 2020; Liu et al., 2020; Mizrahi et al., 2012).

There are many traditional and nontraditional activities that can promote relaxation and stress reduction. These include increasing social supports (e.g., school clubs), physical activity, sports, hobbies, massage, art, music, meditation (e.g., prayers, yoga, tai chi, soothing words or refrains), and autogenic relaxation (combination of visual imagery and body awareness such as breathing rhythm). Although clients and families may have preferred ways to relax (e.g., reading scripture or other family-specific interests) that can be incorporated into therapy, we will review the more general CBT techniques that can be easily implemented in schools and are effective for more significant mental health needs. When performing most of the activities, it may be helpful to ask children and adolescents to close their eyes, as this usually aids focus and concentration. For individuals who choose not to close their eyes, looking off into the distance without focusing on anything will suffice.

Diaphragmatic Breathing

Diaphragmatic breathing has several different names, such as belly breathing and deep breathing. These terms usually refer to focused breathing from the diaphragm, a large, dome-shaped muscle located at the base of the lungs (Cleveland Clinic, n.d.a). The relaxation response elicited by diaphragmatic breathing, a concentrated state of rest and calm, can help reduce physical and psychological distress. Diaphragmatic breathing is sometimes taught through guided scripts that the counselor will read and model until the child can conduct this process on their own. Scripts need to be developmentally appropriate and adapted for the client's vocabulary level. A sample diaphragmatic breathing script can be found in the Appendix, Quick Resource 5.1.

The idea, proposed by Herbert Benson in the 1960s, is to encourage clients to deactivate the "fight or flight" response through controlled breathing and other relaxation strategies (Martin, 2008). As individuals get older, they rely more on chest breathing rather than diaphragmatic breathing because the diaphragm muscle weakens over time, resulting in a lack of sufficient air flow (Medline Plus, n.d.). Thus, subsequent research demonstrates lasting benefits in older age along with stress reduction in anxiety and depression across the lifespan (Martin, 2008). Since diaphragmatic breathing has many benefits—including the proper exchange of oxygen and carbon dioxide, slowing the heartbeat, and reducing blood pressure—it is worthwhile for individuals of all ages to relearn this skill (Harvard Health Publishing, 2020).

In a randomized trial evaluating the efficacy of diaphragmatic breathing relaxation for reducing anxiety, results suggest clinical utility with no negative side effects. Participants were assigned to either a control condition (no training) or the experimental condition (8-week diaphragmatic breathing relaxation training program). Anxiety and four physiological factors were assessed: skin conductivity, peripheral blood flow, heart rate, and breathing rate (Chen et al., 2017). At the end of the program, researchers found statistically significant differences in anxiety for the experimental group across all measures except skin conductivity, with effect sizes ranging from moderate ($d = 0.45$, skin conductivity) to large ($d = 1.90$, heart rate).

Another trial implemented a diaphragmatic breathing course to assess the effect on cognition, affect, and cortisol stress response. The experimental group or breathing intervention group received baseline knowledge and skills for this method of breathing in addition to an 8-week breathing course with coach guidance. The control group received only the baseline skills sessions. The measures utilized were the Positive and Negative Affect Schedule (PANAS) to assess affect (Watson et al., 1988), the Number Cancellation Test (NCT) to assess cognition (Lezak, 1995), and salivary cortisol concentrations. The researchers found small reductions in negative affect and cortisol levels, with similarly small improvements in sustained attention for the intervention group but not the control group (Ma et al., 2017).

Progressive Muscle Relaxation

Progressive muscle relaxation (PMR) is a combination of focused attention on the body, diaphragmatic breathing, and the systematic tightening and loosening of muscle groups throughout one's body. Similar to diaphragmatic breathing, PMR is also taught through guided scripts that the counselor will read and model until the student can conduct this process on their own. Scripts need to be developmentally appropriate and adapted for the client's vocabulary level. A sample PMR script can be found in the Appendix, Quick Resource 5.2.

This technique was established in 1938 by Edmund Jacobson and was originally designed to reduce anxiety and stress (Jacobson, 1938). In a CBT model, practitioners begin by teaching students breathing skills and then discuss the way emotions influence behavior in the body, like anger causing clenched fists. Therapists then demonstrate the difference between bodily tension and relaxation (e.g., "I want you to try to clench your fists as hard as you can for 10 seconds. Now let go of that tension. What do you notice?"). PMR is then explained as a way of using this tension/relaxation contrast throughout the body to relax. While using diaphragmatic breathing, students are taught to move through their bodies and systematically tense and relax their muscles.

In a sample of 4th- and 6th-grade students, PMR and other relaxation methods were tested to evaluate their effect on heart rate, skin temperature, skin conductance level, mood, and physical well-being. The experimenters compared randomized students across four groups: PMR, imagery-based relaxation, listening to neutral stories, and completing arithmetic problems. There effects between the groups were generally small (Lohaus & Klein-Hessling, 2003). Another study showed some reduction in aggressive behavior in 6- to 9-year-olds with emotional/behavioral disorders following PMR compared to a control group. These children were either in day school or treatment programs, and teachers evaluated the frequency of aggressive incidents and ratings with the Child Behavior Checklist (CBCL; Achenbach & Ruffle 2000). Differences at follow-up between the two groups were small on both aggression frequency ($g = 0.13$) and on CBCL scores ($g = 0.13$). Therefore, PMR may be slightly effective for children with emotional and behavioral disorders by proactively reducing arousal to decrease the likelihood of aggressive episodes (Lopata, 2003). Although these effects are small, implementing PMR into CBT is quick and easy; therefore, PMR may be a worthy adjunct to CBT.

PMR also has been shown to decrease various forms of anxiety. Participants in a sample of 387 undergraduate students were randomly assigned to meditation, PMR, or a control group. In the PMR group, nine muscle groups were targeted in their intervention: hands and forearms, upper arms, forehead, eyes/nose/cheeks, jaw/chin/front of neck, back of neck, upper body, legs up with toes pointed down, and legs up with toes pointed up. Stress was induced using a visual stressor, the International Affective Picture System (IAPS; Lang et al., 1995). Differences in state, cognitive, and somatic anxiety were compared between groups before and after the intervention. The results demonstrated small differences across groups for cognitive anxiety and small to moderate effects relative to the control for PMR for state anxiety. On somatic anxiety, all groups improved somewhat, but the PMR group did not improve any more rapidly than the control group, which also experienced intervention gains.

Guided Imagery

Guided imagery involves a concentrated state of relaxation, emphasizes all of the body's senses, and helps students view their thoughts and feelings through a relaxed (rather than anxious or agitated) state (Cleveland Clinic, n.d.b). The term "guided imagery" was coined by David Bresler and Martin Rossman; they defined it as a variety of strategies involving visualization resulting from storytelling, metaphors, or comparable methods (Utay & Miller, 2006). While this practice has been long established in indigenous and religious traditions, psychology did not adopt the concept until the early 1900s in Freud's dream analysis. It appeared in several other theoretical orientations throughout the history of psychology, like when Joseph Wolpe applied the concept to behavior modification therapy in the 1960s. Since then, guided imagery continues to be endorsed by many researchers and practitioners (Utay & Miller, 2006). The technique is simple: Practitioners coach clients to describe a safe place, including sights, smells, sounds, and physical sensations (e.g., sand on one's toes). Often, therapists model guided imagery with their own safe place, allowing the client to experience it with guidance and to select some focal points in their imagery (see the Appendix, Quick Resource 5.3, for a guided imagery script). Like all other scripted counseling resources, there needs to be consideration for developmentally appropriate adaptations in vocabulary and sophistication that match the client's intellectual level and age.

Studies have shown that guided imagery can improve mood and reduce anxiety, stress, smoking, depression, and pain. In a randomized clinical trial, children and adolescents with abdominal pain were randomly assigned to a breathing intervention or a guided imagery with PMR intervention. The intervention was considered successful if by the end of the study they missed no activities and had less than 5 days of pain. At the conclusion of the study, 70% of the children in the guided imagery group met these criteria compared to 14% in the breathing group (Weydert et al., 2006). In one review, the authors suggested that clients utilize more personal images that symbolize their current problems to increase insight and likelihood of behavior change (Varvogli & Darviri, 2011). They noted several applications of guided imagery, including stress reduction (Carter, 2006), preventing smoking relapse (Wynd, 1992), pain management (Antall & Kresevic, 2004; Menzies et al., 2006), treating depression (Lin et al., 2010), and managing stress in overweight adolescents (Weigensberg et al., 2010).

MINDFULNESS

While mindfulness stemmed from Buddhism and Hinduism, mindfulness practice does not need to have a religious or spiritual meaning. It can easily be applied cross-culturally for secular or religious individuals (Brazier, 2013). The earliest incorporation of mindfulness dates back over 4,000 years ago to Pakistan. Modern-day mindfulness practice was pioneered by Jon Kabat-Zinn at the University of

Massachusetts Medical School. He combined his Eastern knowledge of mindfulness with Western science, which caused its popularity to grow exponentially. He created a mindfulness-based therapy program called Mindfulness-Based Cognitive Therapy.

The term "mindfulness" can have a variety of meanings. Most definitions of mindfulness incorporate the systematic development of attention; directing attention to present-moment experiences; cultivating an attitude of acceptance; improving concentration; and developing skills like observing, describing, non-reacting, and non-judging (Zarbock et al., 2015). The original definition of mindfulness as directing one's attention to the present moment was ascribed to Kabat-Zinn (1990).

Mindfulness may include both formal and informal practices. Informal mindfulness is practiced when one slows down routine actions to bring conscious attention to small, daily life activities. An example of informal mindfulness might be a mindful eating exercise in which students focus on a piece of chocolate. The goal of the exercise is to transform an automatic process into a purposeful experience that students can generalize to other behaviors by slowing them down enough to contemplate the purpose of the action (Mathieu, 2009). Students would begin by feeling the weight and texture of the candy in their hand, observing as many details as possible (e.g., rough, smooth, sticky). Next, they smell the candy and then slide their tongue across it to feel its texture. Students might take one small bite and have the candy melt in their mouth while experiencing the candy as though they had never had chocolate in their life. They could then take several small bites, each time focusing on different aspects of the chocolate (e.g., saltiness, sweetness, stickiness). Students and therapists are advised not to rush mindful eating; it might take several minutes (or longer) depending on the chosen stimulus.

In contrast, the formal practice of mindfulness requires consistently dedicating a block of time to focus solely on the breath, body, and mindful movement to pursue a more complex goal (Birtwell et al., 2018). It differs considerably from the small task of focusing on one piece of chocolate. In the formal practice, individuals will set time aside at each meal, every day, to perform a mindful exercise. The more formalized process allows individuals to notice their consumption habits, which could result in more purposeful choices and informed decisions. For example, according to MacDonald (2010), if a person identifies eating habits that seem counterproductive (e.g., eating extremely quickly), they can create a plan to slow their eating process. Slowly and mindfully chewing food could allow someone to feel fuller and eat less.

Other ways to incorporate mindfulness into daily life include listening, walking, yoga, observing, photography, music, exercise, body awareness, technology, parenting, cleaning, and breathing.

The application of mindfulness to psychotherapy practice has been elaborated on and outlined in detail (Pollak et al., 2014; Zarbock et al., 2015). Some popular techniques include yoga, body scan, meditation, breathing exercises, walking meditation, mindful eating, and tai chi. These techniques can have a positive impact on a variety of psychosocial and behavioral problems. The results of a systematic review on sitting meditation in youth underscore the favorable outcomes of meditation practices (Black et al., 2009). Sitting meditation has support for decreasing anxiety, improving absentee periods/rule infractions, lowering externalizing problems and attentional problems, and increasing self-esteem. Median effect sizes for psychosocial/behavioral variables ranged from $d = 0.27$ to $d = 0.70$.

In a meta-analysis on the efficacy of mindfulness-based treatments, Khoury et al. (2013) found large effects on anxiety and depression. For anxiety, 10 pre/post intervention studies and four waitlist control studies produced effect sizes of $g = 0.89$ and $g = 0.96$, respectively. For depression, effect sizes were moderate in five pre/post intervention studies ($g = 0.69$) and eight waitlist control studies ($g = 0.53$).

Nevertheless, some randomized clinical trials have failed to demonstrate a unique effect of mindfulness when compared to an active treatment control. In a randomized controlled trial with 66 participants, researchers compared mindfulness meditation, Argentine tango dance lessons, and a waitlist control (Pinniger et al., 2012). Relative to a waitlist control, mindfulness meditation reduced depression moderately ($d = 0.54$), but so did the tango ($d = 0.50$). Overall stress levels were reduced moderately by the tango ($d = 0.45$), but not by mindfulness. Thus, although mindfulness may evidence some benefit, exercise and concentration on other activities does also; therefore, research is needed comparing it to active control groups.

Mindfulness interventions can provide holistic benefits. For example, mindfulness may help patients manage chronic pain and boost immunity. Additionally, mindfulness may help individuals control challenging health behaviors; supplement treatment for depression, anxiety, and addictive behaviors; improve sustained attention, working memory, and problem-solving abilities; and increase frequency of prosocial behaviors (Creswell, 2017). Although practitioners are reminded that true experimental tests of mindfulness against active control groups are sorely needed, existing evidence supports mindfulness as a useful supplement to CBT.

SUMMARY

This chapter introduced a three-phase approach to psychoeducation to help clients better understand their mental health needs and learn how to exercise control over those struggles. The core component of MI was discussed as a way to facilitate client-based goal setting. Several relaxation techniques were described that may lower stress levels and help students perform activities requiring sustained attention. Mindfulness strategies also were reviewed, including possible benefits and research limitations. The reader is reminded that the strategies covered in this chapter are considered best for clients with mild symptoms or as supplements to the CBT techniques discussed in the next two chapters.

CHAPTER DISCUSSION QUESTIONS

1. Why might psychoeducation improve treatment adherence?
2. How could diaphragmatic breathing be effective on its own, outside of a treatment intervention?
3. Describe the difference between the feelings of tension and relaxation when using progressive muscle relaxation.
4. What aspects of MI differentiate it from traditional CBT?
5. With what cases might a mindfulness approach be useful?
6. In what cases might a mindfulness approach be contraindicated?
7. How might a client's racial, ethnic, or cultural background influence the effectiveness of the interventions discussed in this chapter?

REFERENCES

Achenbach, T. M., & Ruffle, T. M. (2000). The Child Behavior Checklist and related forms for assessing behavioral/emotional problems and competencies. *Pediatrics in Review, 21*, 265–271. https://doi.org/10.1542/pir.21-8-265

Antall, G. F., & Kresevic, D. (2004). The use of guided imagery to manage pain in an elderly orthopaedic population. *Orthopaedic Nursing, 23*(5), 335–340. https://doi.org/10.1097/00006416-200409000-00012

Arnsten, A. F. T. (1998). The biology of being frazzled. *Science, 12*(280), 1711–1712. https://doi.org/10.1126/science.280.5370.1711

Bäuml, J., Froböse, T., Kraemer, S., Rentrop, M., & Pitschel-Walz, G. (2006). Psychoeducation: A basic psychotherapeutic intervention for patients with schizophrenia and their families. *Schizophrenia Bulletin, 32*(Suppl 1), S1–S9. https://doi.org/10.1093/schbul/sbl017

Birtwell, K., Williams, K., van Marwijk, H., Armitage, C. J., & Sheffield, D. (2018). An exploration of formal and informal mindfulness practice and associations with wellbeing. *Mindfulness, 10*, 89–99. https://doi.org/10.1007/s12671-018-0951-y

Black, D. S., Milam, J., & Sussman, S. (2009). Sitting-meditation interventions among youth: A review of treatment efficacy. *Pediatrics, 124*(3), e532–e541. https://doi.org/10.1542/peds.2008-3434

Brazier, C. (2013). Roots of mindfulness. *European Journal of Psychotherapy and Counselling, 15*(2), 127–138. https://doi.org/10.1080/13642537.2013.795336

Brenhouse, H. C., Danese, A., & Grassi-Oliveira, R. (2018). Neuroimmune impacts of early-life stress on development and psychopathology. *Current Topics in Behavioral Neurosciences, 43*, 423–447.

Carter, E. (2006). Pre-packaged guided imagery for stress reduction: Initial results. *Counseling, Psychotherapy, and Health, 2*(2), 27–39.

Chen, Y., Huang, X., Chien, C., & Cheng, J. (2017). The effectiveness of diaphragmatic breathing relaxation training for reducing anxiety. *Perspectives in Psychiatric Care, 53*(4), 329–336. https://doi.org/10.1111/ppc.12184

Cheung, H., Li, W., Lopez, V., Loi, T., & Lee, I. (2007). Psychoeducational preparation of children for surgery: The importance of parental involvement. *Parent Education and Counseling, 65*(1), 34–41. https://doi.org/10.1016/j.pec.2006.04.009

Cleveland Clinic. (n.d.a). *Diaphragmatic breathing*. Retrieved on May 14, 2020, from https://my.clevelandclinic.org/health/articles/9445-diaphragmatic-breathing

Cleveland Clinic. (n.d.b). *Guided imagery*. Retrieved on May 12, 2020, from https://my.clevelandclinic.org/departments/wellness/integrative/treatments-services/guided-imagery

Creswell, J. D. (2017). Mindfulness interventions. *Annual Review of Psychology, 68,* 491–516. https://doi.org/10.1146/annurev-psych-042716-051139

Deffenbacher, J. L., & Stark, R. S. (1992). Relaxation and cognitive-relaxation treatments of general anger. *Journal of Counseling Psychology, 39*(2), 158–167. https://doi.org/10.1037/0022-0167.39.2.158

Ekhtiari, H., Rezapour, T., Aupperle, R. L., & Paulus, M. P. (2017). Neuroscience-informed psychoeducation for addiction medicine: A neurocognitive perspective. *Progress in Brain Research, 235,* 239–264. https://doi.org/10.1016/bs.pbr.2017.08.013

Gayes, L. A., & Steele, R. G. (2014). A meta-analysis of motivational interviewing interventions for pediatric health behavior change. *Journal of Consulting and Clinical Psychology, 82*(3), 521–535. https://doi.org/10.1037/a0035917

Harvard Health Publishing. (2020). *Understanding the stress response: Chronic activation of this survival mechanism impairs health*. Retrieved on June 29, 2020, from www.health.harvard.edu

Jacobson, E. (1938). *Progressive relaxation*. University of Chicago Press.

Joyce-Beaulieu, D. (2020, February). *Counseling applications across MTSS tiers of service*. Presented at the Lee County School Psychologists and Social Workers District In-Service Workshop, Ft. Myers, FL.

Kabat-Zinn, J. (1990). *Full catastrophe living: Using the wisdom of your body and mind to face stress, pain, and illness*. Delacorte Press.

Kessler, R., Schmitt, S., Sauder, T., Stein, F., Yüksel, D., Grotegerd, D., Dannlowski, U., Hahn, T., Dempfle, A., Sommer, J., Steinsträter, O., Nenadic, I., Kircher, T., & Jansen, A. (2020). Long-term neuroanatomical consequences of childhood maltreatment: Reduced amygdala inhibition by medial prefrontal cortex. *Frontiers in Systems Neuroscience, 14,* 28. https://doi.org/10.3389/fnsys.2020.00028

Khoury, B., Lecomte, T., Fortin, G., Masse, M., Therien, P., Bouchard, V., Chapleau, M., Paquin, K., & Hofmann, S. G. (2013). Mindfulness-based therapy: A comprehensive meta-analysis. *Clinical Psychology Review, 33*(6), 763–771. https://doi.org/10.1016/j.cpr.2013.05.005

Lang, P. J., Bradley, M., & Cuthbert, B. (1995). *International Affective Picture System (IAPS): Technical manual and affective ratings*. University of Florida.

Lawrence, P., Fulbrook, P., Somerset, S., & Schulz, P. (2017). Motivational interviewing to enhance treatment attendance in mental health settings: A systematic review and meta-analysis. *Journal of Psychiatric and Mental Health Nursing, 24*(9–10), 699–718. https://doi.org/10.1111/jpm.12420

Lezak, M. (1995). *Neuropsychological assessment* (3rd ed.). Oxford University Press.

Lin, M. F., Hsu, M. C., Chang, H. J., Hsu, Y. Y., Chou, M. H., & Crawford, P. (2010). Pivotal moments and changes in the Bonny method of guided imagery and music for patients with depression. *Journal of Clinical Nursing, 19*(7–8), 1139–1148. https://doi.org/10.1111/j.1365-2702.2009.03140.x

Liu, K., Chen, Y., Wu, D., Lin, R., Wang, Z., & Pan, L. (2020). Effects of progressive muscle relaxation on anxiety and sleep quality in patients with COVID-19. *Complementary Therapies in Clinical Practice, 39*. https://doi.org/10.1016/j.ctcp.2020.101132

Lohaus, A., & Klein-Hessling, J. (2003). Relaxation in children: Effects of extended and intensified training. *Psychology & Health, 18*(2), 237–249. https://doi.org/10.1080/0887044021000057257

Lohaus, A., Klein-Hessling, J., Vogele, C., & Kuhn-Hennighausen, C. (2010). Psychophysiological effects of relaxation training in children. *British Journal of Health Psychology, 6*(2), 197–206. https://doi.org/10.1348/135910701169151

Lopata, C. (2003). Progressive muscle relaxation and aggression among elementary students with emotional or behavioral disorders. *Behavioral Disorders, 28*(2), 162–172. https://doi.org/10.1177/019874290302800203

Ma, X., Yue, Z.-Q., Gong, Z.-Q., Zhang, H., Duan, N.-Y., Shi, Y.-T., Wei, G.-X., & Li, Y.-F. (2017). The effect of diaphragmatic breathing on attention, negative affect and stress in healthy adults. *Frontiers in Psychology, 8*, Article 874. https://doi.org/10.3389/fpsyg.2017.00874

MacDonald, A. (2010, October 19). *Why eating slowly may help you feel full faster.* Harvard Health Publishing. https://www.health.harvard.edu/blog/why-eating-slowly-may-help-you-feel-full-faster-20101019605

Martin, S. (2008). *The power of the relaxation response.* American Psychological Association. Retrieved on March 3, 2020, from https://www.apa.org/monitor/2008/10/relaxation

Mathieu, J. (2009). What should you know about mindful and intuitive eating? *Journal of the Academy of Nutrition and Dietetics, 109*(12), 1982–1986. https://doi.org/10.1016/j.jada.2009.10.023

Maughan, A., & Cicchetti, D. (2003). Impact of child maltreatment and interadult violence on children's emotion regulation abilities and socioemotional adjustment. *Child Development, 73*(5), 1525–1542. https://doi.org/10.1111/1467-8624.00488

Medline Plus. (n.d.). *Aging changes in the lungs.* Retrieved on February 25, 2020, from https://medlineplus.gov/ency/article/004011.htm

Menzies, V., Taylor, A. G., & Bourguignon, C. (2006). Effects of guided imagery on outcomes of pain, functional status, and self-efficacy in persons diagnosed with fibromyalgia. *Journal of Alternative and Complementary Medicine, 12*(1). https://doi.org/10.1089/acm.2006.12.23

Miller, W. R. (1983). Motivational interviewing with problem drinkers. *Behavioral Psychotherapy, 11*(2), 147–172. https://doi.org/10.1017/S0141347300006583

Miller, W. R., & Rollnick, S. (1991). *Motivational interviewing: Preparing people to change addictive behavior.* Guildford Press.

Miller, W. R., & Rollnick, S. (2013). *Motivational interviewing: Helping people change* (3rd ed.). Guilford Press.

Mizrahi, M. C., Reicher-Atir, R., Levy, S., Haramati, S., Wengrower, D., Israeli, E., & Goldin, E. (2012). Effects of guided imagery with relaxation training on anxiety and quality of life among patients with inflammatory bowel disease. *Psychology and Health, 27*(12), 1463–1479. https://doi.org/10.1080/08870446.2012.691169

Norelli, S. K., Long, A., & Krepps, J. M. (2020). *Relaxation techniques*. StatPearls Publishing.

Pechtel, P., & Pizzagalli, D. A. (2011). Effects of early life stress on cognitive and affective function: An integrated review of human literature. *Psychopharmacology, 214*(1), 55–70. https://doi.org/10.1007/s00213-010-2009-2

Pinniger, R., Brown, R. F., Thorsteinsson, E. B., & McKinley, P. (2012). Argentine tango dance compared to mindfulness meditation and a waiting-list control: A randomised trial for treating depression. *Complementary Therapies in Medicine, 20*(6), 377–384. https://doi.org/10.1016/j.ctim.2012.07.003

Pollak, S. M., Pedulla, T., & Siegel, R. D. (2014). *Sitting together: Essential skills for mindfulness-based psychotherapy*. Guilford Publications.

Rollnick, S., & Allison, J. (2004). Motivational interviewing. In N. Heather & T. Stockwell (Eds.), *The essential handbook of treatment and prevention of alcohol problems* (pp. 105–114). Wiley.

Sherin, J. E., & Nemeroff, C. B. (2011). Post-traumatic stress disorder: The neurobiological impact of psychological trauma. *Dialogues in Clinical Neuroscience, 13*(3), 263–278.

Sinha, R. (2008). Chronic stress, drug use, and vulnerability to addiction. *Annals of the New York Academy of Sciences, 1141*, 105–130. https://doi.org/ 10.1196/annals.1441.030

Slavkin, M. L. (2000) The Building Healthy Families model: Psychoeducational practice with children of divorce. *Journal of Divorce & Remarriage, 32*(3-4), 1–17. https://doi.org/10.1300/J087v32n03_01

Thiel, K. J., & Dretsch, M. N. (2011). The basics of the stress response: A historical context and introduction. In D. C. Conrad (Ed.), *The handbook of stress: Neuropsychological effects on the brain* (pp. 3–28). Wiley-Blackwell.

Utay, J., & Miller, M. (2006). Guided imagery as an effective therapeutic technique: A brief review of its history and efficacy research. *Journal of Instructional Psychology, 33*(1), 40–43.

VanBuskirk, K. A., & Wetherell, J. L. (2014). Motivational interviewing with primary care populations: A systematic review and meta-analysis. *Journal of Behavioral Medicine, 37*(4), 768–780. https://doi.org/10.1007/s10865-013-9527-4

Varvogli, L., & Darviri, C. (2011). Stress management techniques: Evidence-based procedures that reduce stress and promote health. *Health Science Journal, 5*, 74–89.

Watson, D., Clark, L. A., & Tellegen, A. (1988). Development and validation of brief measures of positive and negative affect: The PANAS scales. *Journal of Personality and Social Psychology, 54*(6), 1063–1070. https://doi.org/10.1037/0022-3514.54.6.1063

Weigensberg, M. C., Lane, C. J., Winners, O., Wright, T., Nguyen-Rodriguez, S., Goran, M., & Spruijt-Metz (2010). Acute effects of stress-reduction Interactive Guided Imagery[SM] on salivary cortisol in overweight Latino adolescents. *Journal of Alternative and Complementary Medicine, 15*(3), 297–303. https://doi.org/10.1089/acm.2008.0156

Weydert, J. A., Shapiro, D. E., Acra, S. A., Monheim, C. J., Chambers, A. S., & Ball, T. M. (2006). Evaluation of guided imagery as treatment for recurrent abdominal pain in children: A randomized controlled trial. *BMC Pediatrics, 6*, Article 29. https://doi.org/10.1186/1471-2431-6-29

Wynd, C. A. (1992). Relaxation imagery used for stress reduction in the prevention of smoking relapse. *Journal of Advanced Nursing, 17*(3), 294–302. https://doi.org/10.1111/j.1365-2648.1992.tb01907.x

Zaichkowsky, L. B., & Zaichkowsky, L. D. (1983). The effects of a school-based relaxation training program on fourth grade children. *Journal of Clinical Child Psychology, 13*(1), 81–85. https://doi.org/10.1080/15374418409533174

Zarbock, G., Lynch, S., Ammann, A., & Ringer, S. (2015). *Mindfulness for therapists: Understanding mindfulness for professional effectiveness and personal well-being*. Wiley-Blackwell.

Zhang, A., Franklin, C., Jing, S., Bornheimer, L. A., Hai, A. H., Himle, J. A., Kong, D., & Ji, Q. (2019). The effectiveness of four empirically supported psychotherapies for primary care depression and anxiety: A systematic review and meta-analysis. *Journal of Affective Disorders, 245*, 1168–1186. https://doi.org/10.1016/j.jad.2018.12.008

6

Core CBT Components

Part I

LEE N. PURVIS, BRIAN A. ZABOSKI,
AND DIANA JOYCE-BEAULIEU ■

BEHAVIORAL ACTIVATION: INTEGRATING THEORY AND PRACTICE

What Is Behavioral Activation?

Behavioral activation is the "action" component, or guiding principle, of cognitive behavioral therapy (CBT). While therapists may attempt to dispute maladaptive thoughts through logic or reason, the same can be done through changing a client's behavior. Anhedonia and overwhelming feelings of sadness are hallmark features of depressive episodes that decrease pleasurable activity (American Psychiatric Association, 2013). Behavioral activation thus aims to promote engagement in adaptive activities, thereby removing behavioral contingencies that maintain maladaptive behaviors, especially avoidance (Dimidjian et al., 2011). To manage the effects of depression, behavioral activation helps clients recognize avoidant behaviors and identify their core values, promoting their engagement in activities that improve functioning and mood (Lejuez et al., 2011). Behavioral activation employs a host of strategies such as "self-monitoring of activities and mood, activity scheduling/structuring, problem solving, social skills training, hierarchy construction, shaping, reward, and persuasion" (Dimidjian et al., 2011, p. 4).

Behavioral activation can be delivered through a manualized treatment protocol or through non-manualized sessions. The number of behavioral activation and CBT sessions averages around 20 (Martell et al., 2013), but they should be modified to match the implementation parameters within a school. Regarding session length, school-based practitioners might consider 20- to 30-minute sessions. One recommended manualized treatment protocol for children and adolescents is the Brief Behavioral Activation Treatment for Depression (BATD; Lejuez et al., 2011). It condenses the core principles of behavioral activation into, on average, 10 sessions, but it can be lengthened or shortened on a case-by-case basis. The main tenets of BATD include promoting a therapeutic relationship, emphasizing on adaptive domains important to the person (e.g., relationships and academics), values (e.g., supporting friends in need, mastering academic work), activities (e.g., hanging out with a friend after school, studying for a test), daily activity logs for progress monitoring, and troubleshooting treatment barriers (Lejuez et al., 2011). Through BATD, therapists help clients to identify and engage in activities they value by praising action and increasing problem-solving skills that improve treatment adherence.

The clinical efficacy of behavior-based depression treatment was discovered in two seminal studies (Ferster, 1973; Lewinsohn, 1974), which were heavily influenced by research on reinforcement schedules (Herrnstein, 1961). Since then, a plethora of research has been conducted that now supports the significant benefits of behavioral activation in adults with depression. Some studies show that behavioral activation has demonstrated higher effectiveness when the severity level of depression is higher (Webb et al., 2019), and other studies indicate improvements in overall depressive symptomology (McCauley et al., 2016). Behavioral activation emerged as a dominant treatment for depression when researchers found that combining behavioral activation and cognitive restructuring did not lead to better treatment gains than behavioral activation alone (Jacobson et al., 1996). Moreover, researchers continue to show that behavioral activation is equally effective, if not more so, than cognitive restructuring for adolescents (Martin & Oliver, 2019; McCauley et al., 2016; Pass et al., 2016; Webb et al., 2019).

There are several practical considerations when choosing whether to use behavioral activation for adolescents. Higher-order critical thinking skills are still developing in adolescents, which could hinder their ability to benefit from the reflective, insight-driven approaches of cognitive therapy (Johnco et al., 2013), increasing the suitability of behavioral activation. Behavioral activation is easy to adapt to a school-based setting, since the brief session length can accommodate a student's busy academic schedule. Manualized behavioral activation protocols can also be delivered by paraprofessionals with training, supervision, and consultation by school psychologists (Ekers et al., 2011). Behavioral activation may also be particularly helpful for students with comorbid anxiety (Hopko et al., 2004), as anxiety can exacerbate avoidance. Although cognitive strategies are not emphasized within behavioral activation, it does require some cognitive ability. For example, self-reflection is needed for clients to identify their core values and complete daily activity logs (Lejuez et al., 2011).

Like all approaches, behavioral activation is not without its limitations:

1. The literature could benefit from more randomized clinical trials with children and adolescents.

2. The few existing studies include girls from middle to upper socioeconomic status income levels, almost all of them are White. This observation was corroborated in a meta-analysis of behavioral activation treatment studies, only three of which included students of color (Martin & Oliver, 2019). In addition, it also found that most studies suffered from an underrepresentation of males. Consequently, these demographic deficits reduce the ability to generalize findings to diverse student populations.
3. A majority of studies examining the effects of behavioral activation in children and adolescents include case studies or single-subject designs.
4. The meta-analysis revealed that a high number of studies lacked a control group (Martin & Oliver, 2019).

Getting Started: Activity Monitoring

Session 1 of behavioral activation includes psychoeducation on depression, the treatment rationale, and an explanation of the activity monitoring log (Lejuez et al., 2011). The therapist asks students to monitor their activities (however unimportant they may seem) every day until the next session, typically in an activity log (see Quick Resource 6.1 in the Appendix). For instance, a student might log their activity from 8 to 9 a.m. as "sleeping" and from 9 to 10 a.m. as "sleeping," despite having to be in class. In the next session, the clinician reviews the activity log for activities that may be adversely affected by depression; these serve as potential intervention targets. Such activities may include excessive sleeping, eating, and television watching; forgoing activities of daily living (e.g., bathing, brushing teeth); or failing to engage in meaningful activities (e.g., going to school). Conversely, the therapist also pinpoints and praises adaptive behaviors, like going to school, waking up on time, and spending time with friends, while reinforcing a client's participation. Praising the student for their adaptive behaviors and demonstrating the connection between maladaptive activities and depressive symptoms will help to build rapport and encourage a collaborative approach in identifying treatment targets.

Three initial barriers might arise during activity monitoring:

1. For many students, activity monitoring is a new skill. They may be too descriptive in their documentation (so that adding more activities is daunting) or too vague (concealing what the activity entails). Practitioners can minimize confusion by modeling the proper way to log activities. In addition, parents can attend modeling sessions to help children brainstorm, and they can help document ideas throughout the week.
2. Writing can be a source of frustration for some children and adolescents that interferes with activity logging. Text-to-speech devices, sticker

charts to represent activities, or using word processors can help (see Chapter 8 for technology solutions). During the initial visit, clinicians might also informally assess the client's willingness to write.
3. Students with depression may skip or sleep through sessions, and school schedules may interfere with intervention continuity. Remote sessions (with parent assent) can benefit these students, with in-person sessions recommended as later treatment goals.

Identifying Values

After clients can successfully log their behaviors, therapists provide psychoeducation on values. Clients learn that values are ideas that are personally important to them, and that unlike goals, values are not necessarily obtained; rather, they are worked toward (Martell et al., 2013). Common values include interpersonal relationships, work, school, and self-care (Martell et al., 2013). Students then learn that values can be categorized under larger life areas. For a more religious student, interpersonal relationships, work, school, and self-care might all be nested under "spirituality." Next, practitioners customize the student's intervention by helping them express their own values and sorting them into important life domains (Lejuez et al., 2011). The level of subdivision can vary according to the client's development and cognitive ability, but therapists should not overwhelm students with a long list since activities are then generated for each value according to enjoyment and importance.

For most adolescents and adults, a verbal description of values is enough, but visual representations could help younger children and clients with lower cognitive ability. For instance, a therapist might ask a student to rank the last week's top activities they engaged in by their respective life area and to identify their importance and/or enjoyableness. To link life domains, values, and activities, the clinician could provide an example such as, "You've identified spirituality as an aspect of life important to you (domain/life area). A value connected to spirituality is to enhance your faith with the creator (value), so reading a spiritual text for 30 minutes each night (activity) could promote that value."

Behavioral Activation Hierarchy

For homework, the student should continue to add activities under each value. So, if the value is "interpersonal relationships," an initial activity might be "text a friend." Similarly, if a student values "good grades," they might try to study for 5 minutes. The therapist should start with easy activities; the goal is to achieve small successes and then advance to more involved activities each week (Lejuez et al., 2011; Martell et al., 2013). By linking specific behaviors to values in each category, behavioral activation begins to break the cycle of maladaptive thoughts, cognitions, and behaviors. For instance, in the earlier example, behaving consistently with one's values (i.e., texting a friend) can reduce guilt and reinforce positive thoughts about the client's friendship.

Some general advice on activity creation may help practitioners implementing behavioral activation for the first time. Although behavioral activation is tailored to a student's needs, isolation is a common theme for students with depression, and activities that promote social behavior may be helpful. Also, when developing activities, the clinician should solicit detail about the frequency and duration. If the activity is "texting a friend," when and how often will the conversation occur? The collaborative approach between the client and the clinician is indispensable in determining how many activities should be added each week. Progress monitoring and in-session observations, like noticing client mannerisms, reviewing activity logs, and assessing the client's engagement in treatment, can also advise assignment selection. Depending on the severity of the problem behaviors, some clients might tackle multiple tasks each week, while others begin with only one or two. As with most interventions, the clinician will have more responsibility toward the beginning to identify and assign tasks, but this will shift to the student as their insight and motivation improve.

To enhance treatment engagement, support systems can offer additional motivation. In session, counselors are an important ally, providing positive reinforcement for attempted and completed tasks. Additional supports include anyone who has a positive influence and is reliable, typically peers, parents, or teachers. Practitioners should be aware that even with support, students struggle, and students experiencing depression are already self-critical. We recommend that practitioners acknowledge these challenges while avoiding belabored discussions about them—they should spend most of the session advancing goals that reduce depressive symptoms. As treatment engagement increases and students create and practice their list of value-based activities, therapists might consider using a more detailed activity log for progress monitoring and for providing in-session rewards.

Widely Used Progress-Monitoring Systems

Collecting interpretable data on student progress is essential when using behavioral activation. Baseline data establish the severity of depressive symptoms and can reveal underlying comorbid conditions not reported during the initial referral. Additionally, they can reveal motivation levels; insight; and the client's, teachers', and parents' perception of impairment. Throughout the intervention, baseline data will be compared periodically to current functioning to help quantify the student's progress.

Broadband rating scales, which measure many symptoms across different problem behaviors and diagnoses, and narrowband rating scales, which measure a narrower symptom profile, are useful for progress monitoring. Broadband measures include the Behavior Assessment Rating Scale, Third Edition (BASC-3; Reynolds & Kamphaus, 2015); the Brief Inventory for Executive Functioning,

Second Edition (BRIEF-2; Gioia et al., 2015); and the Child Behavior Checklist (CBCL; Achenbach & Edelbrock, 1991). These rating scales have self-, teacher-, and parent-report forms. Examples of narrowband measures include the Beck Depression Inventory, Second Edition (BDI-II; Beck et al., 1996) and the Children's Depression Inventory, Second Edition (CDI-2; Kovacs & Staff, 2011), with the latter comprising self-, teacher-, and parent-report forms. Lastly, examples of self-report, narrowband measures for anxiety and related symptoms include the Revised Children's Manifest Anxiety Scale, Second Edition (RCMAS-2; Reynolds & Richmond, 2008), the Beck Anxiety Inventory (BAI; Beck & Steer, 1990), and the Beck Hopelessness Scale (BHS; Beck & Steer, 1988). These measures are also useful postintervention to assess longer-term treatment gains.

Progress monitoring for educational (e.g., grades, office-discipline referrals) and clinical (e.g., BDI-II) outcomes over time should be collected from the client, teacher, and/or parents (Borntrager & Lyon, 2015). With multiple raters across multiple settings, practitioners can personalize interventions (e.g., address anxiety primarily present during test taking), predict discrepant results (e.g., behavior ratings will not improve much at home where there is less structure), and show symptom changes across raters/settings over time (De Los Reyes et al., 2015). Additionally, as children and adolescents are more likely to underestimate the impact of depression, progress monitoring might also capture a student's developing insight (Creswell et al., 2014; Hunt et al., 2003). These data can be used to provide feedback to the student, teachers, and parents and to guide clinical decision-making (Creswell et al., 2014).

Clinicians should accommodate students as needed and select measures that fit a client's age and cognitive ability. For example, they can read items aloud to younger children and cognitively impaired adolescents. Scaling questions can also help; for example, *On a scale of 1 to 5, how would you rate your depression?* (Sklare, 2014). Scaling questions provide a point of comparison to the previous sessions and encourage students to speak candidly about their feelings. For older students, graphs of their data could maintain commitment to treatment by demonstrating accomplishments and normalizing the typical ups and downs of success. Requesting that students maintain a confidential folder of these session materials can facilitate review of assignments and improve organizational skills.

COGNITIVE RESTRUCTURING: INTEGRATING THEORY AND PRACTICE

What Is Cognitive Restructuring?

According to Aaron Beck (2005), automatic thoughts, or thoughts that appear in consciousness absent one's control, are associated with emotional and behavioral responses. People are unaware of most of these thoughts, and since they usually align with their core beliefs, the resulting behaviors are adaptive. For example, an academically oriented student may receive an assignment, automatically think,

"This will be tough, but I can do it," and then work on the task. However, some people with internalizing disorders, like depression, evidence automatic thoughts that are irrational and not fact-based. These distorted thoughts increase the likelihood of negative affect and maladaptive behaviors (Rnic et al., 2016). In the prior example with the academically oriented student, if the automatic thought were, "This is impossible!" then this student may procrastinate or refuse to do the assignment. Refer to Quick Resource 6.2 in the Appendix for a list of cognitive distortions and examples.

Cognitive restructuring is a core CBT component that challenges distorted thinking. Clients first identify the illogical beliefs, attitudes, and meanings they affix to situations and experiences in the environment (Edwards, 1990). Then, to develop healthy beliefs and action plans, the therapist helps the student evaluate the thoughts objectively (Rosenberg et al., 2011). Cognitive restructuring is frequently used when treating anxiety, depression, and trauma. Cognitive restructuring also has applications for neurodevelopmental disorders, like attention-deficit/hyperactivity disorder and autism spectrum disorder. Most insight and action therapies use cognitive restructuring as a core component, including trauma-focused CBT, dialectical behavior therapy (DBT), rational emotive behavior therapy, and gestalt therapy.

Parker et al. (2016) emphasize a four-part structure in cognitive restructuring. First is psychoeducation on how thoughts, feelings, and behaviors interact. During the second stage, the student's mastery of psychoeducation is enhanced through identification of their own thoughts, feelings, and behaviors and how they connect. In the third stage, clinicians provide psychoeducation on automatic thoughts. With insight from the first three stages and a strong therapeutic alliance, clients can engage in the fourth stage, challenging maladaptive, automatic thoughts. An alternative, six-stage cognitive restructuring model includes assessing how the irrational belief was acquired and ascertaining whether maladaptive emotions stem from an automatic thought, an underlying belief, or a felt meaning (Edwards, 1990). Regardless of the model used, cognitive restructuring primarily focuses on disputing irrational thoughts to alter negative affect, thereby increasing engagement in positive behaviors. This section will focus on cognitive restructuring techniques commonly applied within Beck's cognitive therapy model (see Chapter 2).

Evaluating the Evidence

A mixture of techniques is used to enhance the effectiveness of cognitive restructuring, including evaluating the evidence, thought logs, adapted guided imagery, and Socratic questioning, as well as vignettes, role plays, and concrete examples. The "evaluating the evidence" technique was first used within CBT and is also a core component of DBT called "Checking the Facts" (Linehan, 1993). Checking the Facts allows clients to evaluate the accuracy of their beliefs by identifying the distorted belief and then providing counterevidence. For example, a person may think "No one likes being around me," leading to feelings of sadness. The clinician would then ask them to recognize the feeling but challenge it by providing factual evidence to support the thought. After repeated practice, clients learn how to defend against emotional reasoning (the fallacy of feeling that something is true without having any facts to support it).

Guided Imagery Application in Cognitive Restructuring

Guided imagery (as described in Chapter 5) is often used as a relaxation strategy by having the client visualize a peaceful setting. However, it also can be adapted to facilitate cognitive restructuring. The adapted version would ask the client to recall a specific event with therapist guidance. As stated by Tusek et al. (1997), guided imagery uses "the power of thought to influence psychological and physiological states" (p. 172). Practitioners use it to relieve the discomfort of depressive symptoms and to interrupt rumination (unwanted and repetitive thoughts about a problem; Apóstolo & Kolcaba, 2009). As an example, a client may think, "no one likes being around me," which could lead to self-imposed social isolation. A school psychologist would ask a scaling question to obtain a baseline (e.g., "How sad does the thought make you feel on a scale of 1 to 10?") and then encourage the client to think of a recent positive interaction they had with a peer. The clinician can also provide scenarios to aid recollection, such as lunch, recess, or extracurricular activities. The client closes their eyes and describes the setting in detail while taking particular note of their positive feelings. After they finish the technique, the clinician would ask the same scaling question as before. Thus, using this technique, the client disputed their thought by recalling evidence that directly challenged it.

Thought Records

Students use thought logs/records to document and refute negative automatic thoughts and feelings connected to a triggering event, replacing them with more balanced thinking (Josefowitz, 2017). A thought log provides another visual representation of cognitive restructuring techniques, such as checking the facts, and has even demonstrated improved use through guided imagery as described earlier (Josefowitz, 2017). Documentation through thought logs should be used primarily in adolescents and adults due to the difficulties younger children display when attempting to recall emotions connected to negative thinking (Curry & Reinecke, 2003). However, this technique may be modified for younger children by using more imaginative words like "thought monsters" or "thought bubbles" and providing concrete visual examples to reinforce learning (Garber et al., 2016). Initially, clients should not use thought records to challenge negative thoughts; rather, they should merely identify them and the related emotions. After achieving sustained mastery of recognizing automatic thoughts and their effects on behavior, they can then use thought logs to challenge negative thinking.

Socratic Questioning

CBT borrows a technique from the Greek philosopher Socrates, who was famous for the Socratic method, an approach that decomposes a challenging problem into a series of questions that, when answered, reveal a solution. Socratic questioning distinguishes regular conversations from therapeutic ones. It requires the clinician to ask probing questions, engage in active listening, reflect statements back to the client, and then synthesize questions that require further reflection (Padesky, 1993). Examples of questions that synthesize information and encourage further reflection include, "What do you believe your decision to finish your homework instead of play video games says about your work ethic?"; "How would you know when you're feeling upset?"; "If your friend Justin went through a breakup like you're going through, would you tell him he's weak if he misses her?"

In CBT, Socratic questioning is used to increase clients' insight into their distorted thoughts and help them arrive to answers on their own. Sklare (2014) proposes that treatment can be enhanced when clients recognize their own irrational thoughts rather than being told directly by the therapist. Additionally, it can help children and adolescents identify the function of their behaviors, pinpoint triggers that increase maladaptive emotions and thoughts, and recognize physiological effects of stress or anxiety. This method also allows the student to reframe their thoughts in more beneficial ways.

The following is an example of Socratic questioning in a larger therapeutic dialog. Notable micro skills (Chapter 3) and foundational skills (Chapter 5) are indicated in parentheses.

> Therapist: Tell me about the last time you were upset. *(open-ended question)*
> Client: Yesterday, I was playing basketball with my friend Ethan and he passed the ball to me, but I wasn't looking, and it hit me in the mouth. I was really mad.
> T: Oh wow, I bet that did hurt. *(empathy)* What did you do next? *(probing question)*
> C: I took a few deep breaths and continued playing the game.
> T: So, taking some deep breaths after being hit by the ball allowed you to continue to play the game? *(reflect statement back to client in context of therapy goals)*
> C: I guess so, and I figured Ethan didn't mean to hit me.
> T: Hmm, so by implementing a coping strategy, you were able to pause and determine how you were going to respond to the situation that would result in the best possible outcome? *(bridging statement)*
> C: Oh yeah, I didn't even realize I practiced one of our calm down techniques.

T: Exactly! Good job! *(acknowledgment statements)* Now imagine a similar incident like this happens in the future at school with someone you didn't like hitting you with the basketball. How would you respond then? *(probing question)*

C: Hmm . . . I'd probably need to do more than take a deep breath because I'd want to hit that guy back with the ball.

T: So you'd be really angry with him. *(reflecting statement)* Then what would happen if you hit him? *(probing question)*

C: I'd probably get suspended.

T: Yeah, and we wouldn't want that to happen. You mentioned earlier you'd need to do more than deep breathing. Sounds to me like you'd want to respond in a different way so you wouldn't get into trouble. What else would help you reduce your anger in that moment? *(probing question)*

C: I may want to take a break or count backward from 10.

T: Those are both very good options that wouldn't get you in trouble. I have to admit, I'm extremely proud of you and your ability to identify strategies to reduce your anger which would allow you to respond in a way that wouldn't get you in trouble. *(summary statement)*

In this example, the therapist uses open-ended questions, empathy, and reflection to help the student acknowledge their positive behavior and consider how similar behavior may help in the future. Moreover, the therapist encourages the client to consider the counseling tools they learned and to think about how to apply those tools to a new situation.

Assessing Cognitive Distortions

Rating scales measuring disordered thinking are less common than those measuring behavioral activation. Two rating scales highlighted in the literature include the How I Think Questionnaire (HIT-Q; Barriga et al., 2001) and the Children's Negative Cognitive Errors Questionnaire—Revised (CNCEQ-R; Maric et al., 2011). These measures are not recommended for progress monitoring due to their length, but using them as preintervention and postintervention measures could be advantageous for identifying shifts in thinking. Additional measures that may provide further insight into depressive and anxious symptomology include the CDI-2, RCMAS-2, BAI, and BHS discussed earlier in the chapter.

Efficacy of Cognitive Restructuring

At present, the benefits of cognitive restructuring are established for adults, but more research is needed with children. One study on older adults analyzed the relationship between cognitive impairment, cognitive restructuring skills, and design fluency (Johnco et al., 2013). When categorized into poor- and good-quality acquisition of cognitive restructuring skills, those in the poor quality group demonstrated greater cognitive impairment ($g = 0.86$) and a higher number of errors on a design fluency task ($g = 0.88$; Johnco et al., 2013). In a non-randomized study, cognitive restructuring, behavioral activation, and core belief strategies were used within 43 CBT groups with roughly nine adults per group ($N = 312$) across 14 sessions. Decreases on the BDI-II from Session 1 to Session 14 were noted for patients with severe depression ($d = -1.59$) and moderate depression ($d = -1.44$; Hawley et al., 2017).

In children/adolescents, the effects of cognitive restructuring are often investigated as part of larger CBT protocols. For example, Shirk et al. (2013) treated 44 adolescents with depression with a 12-session manualized protocol containing three modules: cognitive (identify negative thoughts and related feelings), behavioral (stress management and implementation of productive and pleasurable activities), and interpersonal (individually tailored to the needs of the individual, ranging from anger management to social anxiety). Their manualized treatment protocol (including cognitive restructuring) decreased depressive symptoms by 20 points on a measure of depression. Additionally, they found that changes in cognitive distortions throughout treatment predicted lower depressive symptoms after treatment even controlling for early improvement ($\beta = 0.28$). The authors conclude that "cognitive distortions are a pivotal change mechanism in CBT for adolescent depression" (p. 320), highlighting the potential utility of cognitive restructuring in CBT protocols.

Despite evidence suggesting that cognitive restructuring is effective in adults and likely effective in adolescents, it is not clear whether it outperforms behavioral activation. A school-based study with 40 adolescent girls with depression compared behavioral, cognitive, and relational components of CBT (e.g., therapeutic alliance and group synergy; Arora et al., 2019). School-based treatment was delivered in 20 group sessions and 2 individual sessions over 11 weeks. The authors found that behavioral interventions were associated with higher decreases in depression scores ($\beta = 0.18$) than cognitive interventions ($\beta = 0.06$). When age was used a moderator between intervention components and depressive symptoms, younger girls benefited more from the behavioral ($\beta = -0.22$) component; and contrary to their hypotheses, older students did not benefit more from the cognitive components ($\beta = 0.10$, $p > 0.05$). Nevertheless, while preliminary studies suggest that behavioral activation may have stronger literature support, cognitive techniques have an important place in a therapist's skillset. Thus, we recommend that practitioners consider augmenting behavioral activation with cognitive restructuring to further customize CBT to students within diverse school environments.

CASE STUDY: KJ, THE KID EVERYBODY WANTED TO BE

KJ is an 11-year-old American Indian male enrolled in Y.A. Middle School as a 6th grader. Prior to the current school year, KJ would have been considered athletic, smart, and outgoing according to his friends and teachers. Since elementary school, KJ has been involved in a range of extracurricular activities, including the robotics club and student government, and is an active church member. Academically, KJ's grades on coursework were always in the A-range, and he performed well on standardized tests, but since the start of the new academic year, he started to exhibit atypical behavior. The shift in behavior was apparent to his peers when he decided not to run for student government office (the previous year he ran unopposed). He also quit the robotics club, he now eats his lunch in the library, and his grades have dropped to Cs and Ds.

Due to the drastic decline in KJ's overall functioning, his teacher referred him to the school counselor, Ms. Lewis, for a skills group she was forming with 6th-grade boys. After four sessions, KJ's counselor decided to refer him to the school psychologist, Mr. Lambeau, for individualized sessions since he showed no marked improvement, and the group mainly worked on academic and motivational skills. During Mr. Lambeau's first session (rapport building and a semistructured interview), KJ mainly responded in monosyllabic words until asked about his family. He began to cry, and instead of probing further, Mr. Lambeau validated his emotions and sat with him until he wanted to continue. KJ reported that his parents got a divorce 1 week before school started. KJ also shared that after failing his first two tests in the school year, he gave up trying to study, considers himself a failure, and is embarrassed to interact with his friends because of how he may be judged.

In the next session, KJ reported feeling excited to see Mr. Lambeau because he was able to safely disclose triggering events in his life. After validating and reflecting KJ's mood, Mr. Lambeau provided treatment rationales for behavioral activation and cognitive restructuring. KJ readily understood the information and over the next few sessions responded positively to behavioral activation strategies and started sitting with his friends at lunch again. His grades rebounded to all Cs on his next report card. Although Mr. Lambeau praised KJ's improvements, he thought cognitive restructuring techniques would yield more significant gains. When Mr. Lambeau was attempting to help increase KJ's insight into cognitive distortions fueling his maladaptive behaviors, KJ exhibited frustration when Mr. Lambeau used Socratic questioning and even walked out of a session when probed further. Mr. Lambeau attempted to utilize the "Check the Facts" strategy, but the same frustration was visible. Now, Mr. Lambeau does not know how to proceed without breaking rapport.

SUMMARY

Two core CBT skills for adolescents with depression are behavioral activation and cognitive restructuring. Behavioral activation addresses behavioral contingencies that maintain depressed behaviors (Dimidjian et al., 2011), and cognitive restructuring identifies and replaces negative cognitions with more adaptive beliefs (Rosenberg et al., 2011). There is a growing body of research validating these techniques in children and adolescents, with stronger evidence supporting behavioral activation. Implementing these services in schools with help from paraprofessionals can increase access to mental health services and include more people of color and lower socioeconomic status. Furthermore, studies could benefit from treatment fidelity checks, frequent progress monitoring to establish stronger clinical conclusions, and multiple treatment approaches. Refer to Quick Resources 6.3 and 6.4 in the Appendix for parent psychoeducation handouts describing behavioral activation and cognitive restructuring.

CHAPTER DISCUSSION QUESTIONS

1. What are some of the cognitive behavioral treatment options for a person presenting with depression?
2. What are the potential barriers to the utilization of cognitive restructuring in children and adolescents?
3. What aspects of behavioral activation should be standardized? Which can be altered to fit the client's characteristics?
4. Would behavioral activation or cognitive restructuring be more appropriate for a person with above-average intelligence but limited social engagement? Provide support for your answer.
5. Could any cognitive distortions be attributed to demographic characteristics (e.g., race, gender, age)? Why?
6. What are some treatment considerations in behavioral activation and cognitive restructuring specific to individuals from disenfranchised communities?
7. How involved should parents be in the cognitive behavioral treatment process? What environmental factors should be considered in this decision?

REFERENCES

Achenbach, T. M., & Edelbrock, C. (1991). *Manual for the Child Behavior Checklist and 1991 Profile*. University of Vermont Department of Psychiatry.

American Psychiatric Association. (2013). *Diagnostic and statistical manual of mental disorders* (5th ed.). https://doi.org/10.1176/appi.books.9780890425596

Apóstolo, J. L. A., & Kolcaba, K. (2009). The effects of guided imagery on comfort, depression, anxiety, and stress of psychiatric inpatients with depressive disorders. *Archives of Psychiatric Nursing, 23*(6), 403–411. https://doi.org/10.1016/j.apnu.2008.12.003

Arora, P. G., Baker, C. N., Marchette, L. K., & Stark, K. D. (2019). Components analyses of a school-based cognitive behavioral treatment for youth depression. *Journal of Clinical Child & Adolescent Psychology, 48*(Supp 1), S180–S193. https://doi.org/10.1080/15374416.2017.1280800

Barriga, A. Q., Gibbs, J. C., Potter, G., & Liau, A. K. (2001). *The How I Think Questionnaire manual*. Research Press.

Beck, A. T. (2005). The current state of cognitive therapy: A 40-year retrospective. *Archives of General Psychiatry, 62*(9), 953–959. https://doi.org/10.1001/archpsyc.62.9.953

Beck, A. T., & Steer, R. A. (1988). *Manual for the Beck Hopelessness Scale*. Psychological Corporation.

Beck, A. T., & Steer, R. A. (1990). *Manual for the Beck Anxiety Inventory*. Psychological Corporation.

Beck, A. T., Steer, R. A., & Brown, G. K. (1996). *Manual for the Beck Depression Inventory-II*. Psychological Corporation.

Borntrager, C., & Lyon, A. R. (2015). Monitoring client progress and feedback in school-based mental health. *Cognitive and Behavioral Practice, 22*(1), 74–86. https://doi.org/10.1016/j.cbpra.2014.03.007

Creswell, C., Waite, P., & Cooper, P. J. (2014). Assessment and management of anxiety disorders in children and adolescents. *Archives of Disease in Childhood, 99*(7), 674–678. http://dx.doi.org/10.1136/archdischild-2013-303768

Curry, J. F., & Reinecke, M. A. (2003). Modular therapy for adolescents with major depression. In M. A. Reinecke, F. M. Dattilio, & A. Freeman (Eds.), *Cognitive therapy with children and adolescents: A casebook for clinical practice* (pp. 95–128). Guilford Press.

De Los Reyes, A., Augenstein, T. M., Wang, M., Thomas, S. A., Drabick, D. A., Burgers, D. E., & Rabinowitz, J. (2015). The validity of the multi-informant approach to assessing child and adolescent mental health. *Psychological Bulletin, 141*(4), 858–900. https://doi.org/10.1037/a0038498

Dimidjian, S., Barrera Jr, M., Martell, C., Muñoz, R. F., & Lewinsohn, P. M. (2011). The origins and current status of behavioral activation treatments for depression. *Annual Review of Clinical Psychology, 7*, 1–38. https://doi.org/10.1146/annurev-clinpsy-032210-104535

Edwards, D. J. (1990). Cognitive therapy and the restructuring of early memories through guided imagery. *Journal of Cognitive Psychotherapy, 4*(1), 33–50.

Ekers, D., Richards, D., McMillan, D., Bland, J. M., & Gilbody, S. (2011). Behavioural activation delivered by the non-specialist: Phase II randomised controlled trial. *British Journal of Psychiatry, 198*(1), 66–72. https://doi.org/10.1192/bjp.bp.110.079111

Ferster, C. B. (1973). A functional analysis of depression. *American Psychologist, 28*(10), 857–870. https://doi.org/10.1037/h0035605

Garber, J., Frankel, S. A., & Herrington, C. G. (2016). Developmental demands of cognitive behavioral therapy for depression in children and adolescents: Cognitive, social, and emotional processes. *Annual Review of Clinical Psychology, 12*(1), 181–216. https://doi.org/10.1146/annurev-clinpsy-032814-112836

Gioia, G. A., Isquith, P. K., Guy, S. C., Kenworthy, L. (2015). *Behavior Rating Inventory of Executive Function®, Second Edition (BRIEF®2)*. PAR Inc.

Hawley, L. H., Padesky, C. A., Hollon, S. D., Mancuso, E., Laposa, J. M., Brozina, K., & Segal, Z. V. (2017). Cognitive-behavioral therapy for depression using mind over mood: CBT skill use and differential symptom alleviation. *Behavior Therapy, 48*(1), 29–44. http://dx.doi.org/10.1016/j.beth.2016.09.003

Herrnstein, R. J. (1961). Relative and absolute strength of response as a function of frequency of reinforcement. *Journal of the Experimental Analysis of Behavior, 4*(3), 267–272. https://doi.org/10.1901/jeab.1961.4-267

Hopko, D. R., Lejuez, C. W., & Hopko, S. D. (2004). Behavioral activation as an intervention for coexistent depressive and anxiety symptoms. *Clinical Case Studies, 3*(1), 37–48. https://doi.org/10.1177/1534650103258969

Hunt, M., Auriemma, J., & Cashaw, A. C. (2003). Self-report bias and underreporting of depression on the BDI-II. *Journal of Personality Assessment, 80*(1), 26–30. https://doi.org/10.1207/S15327752JPA8001_10

Jacobson, N. S., Dobson, K. S., Truax, P. A., Addis, M. E., Koerner, K., Gollan, J. K., Gortner, E., & Prince, S. E. (1996). A component analysis of cognitive-behavioral treatment for depression. *Journal of Consulting and Clinical Psychology, 64*(2), 295–304. https://doi.org/10.1037//0022-006x.64.2.295

Johnco, C., Wuthrich, V. M., & Rapee, R. M. (2013). The role of cognitive flexibility in cognitive restructuring skill acquisition among older adults. *Journal of Anxiety Disorders, 27*(6), 576–584. https://doi.org/10.1016/j.janxdis.2012.10.004

Josefowitz, N. (2017). Incorporating imagery into thought records: Increasing engagement in balanced thoughts. *Cognitive and Behavioral Practice, 24*(1), 90–100. https://doi.org/10.1016/j.cbpra.2016.03.005

Kovacs, M., & Staff, M. (2011). *Children's Depression Inventory 2nd edition (CDI-2) technical manual*. Multi-Health Systems.

Lejuez, C. W., Hopko, D. R., Acierno, R., Daughters, S. B., & Pagoto, S. L. (2011). Ten year revision of the brief behavioral activation treatment for depression: Revised treatment manual. *Behavior Modification, 35*(2), 111–161. https://doi.org/10.1177/0145445510390929

Lewinsohn, P. M. (1974). A behavioral approach to depression. In R. J. Friedman & M. M. Katz (Eds.), *The psychology of depression: Contemporary theory and research*. John Wiley & Sons.

Linehan, M. (1993). *Skills training manual for treating borderline personality disorder*. Guilford Press.

Maric, M., Heyne, D. A., van Widenfelt, B. M., & Westenberg, P. M. (2011). Distorted cognitive processing in youth: The structure of negative cognitive errors and their associations with anxiety. *Cognitive Therapy and Research, 35*, 11–20. https://doi.org/10.1007/s10608-009-9285-3

Martell, C. R., Dimidjian, S., & Herman-Dunn, R. (2013). *Behavioral activation for depression: A clinician's guide*. Guilford Press.

Martin, F., & Oliver, T. (2019). Behavioral activation for children and adolescents: A systematic review of progress and promise. *European Child & Adolescent Psychiatry, 28*(4), 427–441. https://doi.org/10.1007/s00787-018-1126-z

McCauley, E., Gudmundsen, G., Schloredt, K., Martell, C., Rhew, I., Hubley, S., & Dimidjian, S. (2016). The adolescent behavioral activation program: Adapting behavioral activation as a treatment for depression in adolescence. *Journal of Clinical Child & Adolescent Psychology, 45*(3), 291–304. https://doi.org/10.1080/15374416.2014.979933

Padesky, C. A. (1993, September 24). *Socratic questioning: Changing minds or guiding discovery?* Keynote address, European Congress of Behavioural and Cognitive Therapies, London, England. https://padesky.com/newpad/wp-content/uploads/2012/11/socquest.pdf

Parker, J., Zaboski, B., & Joyce-Beaulieu, D. (2016). School-based cognitive-behavioral therapy for an adolescent presenting with ADHD and explosive anger: A case study. *Contemporary School Psychology, 20*(4), 356–369. https://doi.org/10.1007/s40688-016-0093-y

Pass, L., Whitney, H., & Reynolds, S. (2016). Brief behavioral activation for adolescent depression: Working with complexity and risk. *Clinical Case Studies, 15*(5), 360–375. https://doi.org/10.1177/1534650116645402

Reynolds, C. R., & Kamphaus, R. W. (2015). *Behavior Assessment System for Children–Third Edition (BASC-3)*. Pearson.

Reynolds, C. R., & Richmond, B. O. (2008). *Revised Children's Manifest Anxiety Scale, Second Edition (RCMAS-2)*. Western Psychological Services.

Rnic, K., Dozois, D. J., & Martin, R. A. (2016). Cognitive distortions, humor styles, and depression. *Europe's Journal of Psychology, 12*(3), 348–362. https://doi.org/10.5964/ejop.v12i3.1118

Rosenberg, H. J., Jankowski, M. K., Fortuna, L. R., Rosenberg, S. D., & Mueser, K. T. (2011). A pilot study of a cognitive restructuring program for treating posttraumatic disorders in adolescents. *Psychological Trauma: Theory, Research, Practice, and Policy, 3*(1), 94–99.

Shirk, S. R., Crisostomo, P. S., Jungbluth, N., & Gudmundsen, G. R. (2013). Cognitive mechanisms of change in CBT for adolescent depression: Associations among client involvement, cognitive distortions, and treatment outcome. *International Journal of Cognitive Therapy, 6*(4), 311–324. https://doi.org/10.1521/ijct.2013.6.4.311

Sklare, G. B. (2014). *Brief counseling that works: A solution-focused therapy approach for school counselors and other mental health professionals*. Corwin Press.

Tusek, D. L., Church, J. M., Strong, S. A., Grass, J. A., & Fazio, V. W. (1997). Guided imagery: A significant advance in the care of patients undergoing elective colorectal surgery. *Diseases of the Colon & Rectum, 40*(2), 172–178. https://doi.org/10.1007/BF02054983

Webb, C. A., Stanton, C. H., Bondy, E., Singleton, P., Pizzagalli, D. A., & Auerbach, R. P. (2019). Cognitive versus behavioral skills in CBT for depressed adolescents: Disaggregating within-patient versus between-patient effects on symptom change. *Journal of Consulting and Clinical Psychology, 87*(5), 484–490. https://doi.org/10.1037/ccp0000393

7

Core CBT Components

Part II

ERIN K. REID, LESLIE K. TAYLOR, KELLY N. BANNEYER,
JOSE DOMINGUEZ, GARY LIU, LAUREL L. WILLIAMS,
BRIAN A. ZABOSKI, SOPHIE C. SCHNEIDER,
AND ERIC A. STORCH ■

EXPOSURE THERAPY: INTEGRATING THEORY AND PRACTICE

Cognitive behavioral therapy (CBT) with exposure and response prevention is a first-line treatment for anxiety and obsessive-compulsive disorder (OCD) in children and adolescents (Abramowitz et al., 2005; Bergez et al., 2020; Connolly & Bernstein, 2007; McGuire et al., 2015; Wang et al., 2017). In a meta-analysis of treatments for childhood anxiety disorders, CBT and medication resulted in greater reductions in anxiety symptoms compared to pill placebo and waitlist conditions (Wang et al., 2017), with a clear advantage of CBT relative to antidepressant medications for school-aged children with OCD (McGuire et al., 2015). CBT has demonstrated safety and therapist and patient acceptability (Schneider et al., 2020), including fewer adverse events with CBT than medications and fewer dropouts with CBT than other treatments (Johnco et al., 2020; Wang et al., 2017). CBT involves several core treatment components: exposure and response prevention, cognitive therapy, and psychoeducation (Peris et al., 2020).

Exposure therapy is the central component with therapeutic benefit compared to other techniques such as psychoeducation, cognitive strategies, and relaxation (Higa-McMillan et al., 2016). Exposure therapy encourages youth to engage with their specific distress/anxiety-provoking stimuli without engaging in avoidant, ritualistic, and safety behaviors in a systematic and gradual fashion. Avoidant behavior involves excessive efforts to prevent experiencing an anxiety-provoking trigger like social events/interactions, classroom activities, unfamiliar situations, unsanitary areas, storms, needles, or insects. Primarily in OCD but also in other anxiety conditions, ritualistic behaviors, or compulsions, are performed in response to distress/anxiety-provoking triggers, such as excessive handwashing in students with contamination obsessions. Finally, safety behaviors refer to actions that temporarily relieve anxiety, such as asking for reassurance and engaging in situations only if certain conditions are met (e.g., together with a parent, having a cellphone available in case of emergency). Across all theoretical models of exposure therapy, safety behaviors weaken the effect of the intervention.

The goals of this chapter are to describe the theoretical background and central components of exposure therapy and to explain how school-based mental health (SMH) professionals can implement exposure therapy. First, the theoretical framework for exposure therapy is presented and the central components of exposure therapy in school-based practice are described. Second, principles of cognitive restructuring and how to apply them in the context of exposure therapy are discussed. Third, special considerations for implementing trauma-informed exposure therapy in the schools are reviewed. Lastly, a case report describing anxiety treatment in a school setting is presented.

Theoretical Framework

The theoretical underpinnings for exposure therapy have evolved over time. This section will briefly review the following models: systemic desensitization, habituation, and inhibitory learning. First, Wolpe popularized systematic desensitization in the mid-1900s (Wolpe, 1958). In systematic desensitization, individuals are taught relaxation strategies and then asked to engage in imaginal exposures, a type of exposure that is pictured in one's mind (for example, tripping in a crowded lunchroom). Systematic desensitization was theorized to improve anxiety through reciprocal inhibition, a state of relaxation in the presence of progressively difficult imaginal exposures (Wolpe, 1958). Although early studies showed that relaxation and exposure were both required to reduce anxiety (e.g., Lang & Lazovik, 1963), subsequent studies found that relaxation was not necessary for anxiety reduction (Dawson & McMurray, 1978; Gillan & Rachman, 1974) and may even have had detrimental effects on intervention outcomes.

A subsequent theoretical framework, the habituation model (Lader & Wing, 1966), arose from the idea that exposure without relaxation was sufficient for reducing anxiety. This model purports that exposure is effective when (a) the fear response is activated, (b) avoidant behaviors are minimized, and (c) anxiety reduction occurs within and between exposures (Benito & Walther, 2015). For instance, habituation predicts that a child who is fearful of germs on doorknobs can repeatedly touch them without avoidance to reduce their anxiety. Through repeated practice, anxiety would decrease within a single session and between sessions.

Expanding on habituation, emotional processing theory (EPT) combines it with the concept of new learning (Foa & Kozak, 1986). In EPT, new learning occurs when "fear structures" are replaced with non-fear structures through repeated exposures (Foa & Kozak, 1986; Foa & McLean, 2016). Specifically, proponents of EPT claim that levels of initial fear activation, within-session habituation, and between-session habituation predict fear reduction and that within-session habituation must precede between-session habituation (Foa & Kozak, 1986). Research findings on these tenets of EPT are inconsistent and provide minimal support for its components as predictors of symptom reduction (see Craske et al., 2008). Indeed, recent studies found that a decrease in anxiety within and between sessions is not a necessary condition for anxiety reduction (Peterman et al., 2019).

Inhibitory learning is a contemporary theoretical model that addresses shortcomings in prior theories of exposure therapy. For example, the inhibitory learning model states that the original conditioned anxiety response (doorknobs → anxiety) will never completely extinguish. Instead, a competing non-anxious response to the same feared situation (doorknobs → no anxiety) inhibits the original response (Craske et al., 2008, 2014). Thus, the original fear pathway (doorknobs → anxiety) is still there; it is just inhibited through exposure therapy. This implies that if a child does not continue to practice exposures that strengthen the adaptive learning (i.e., that doorknobs → no anxiety), then the original fear response can return (Hezel & Simpson, 2019).

Another key tenet of inhibitory learning is expectancy violation. Exposures are most effective when there is a large discrepancy between the expected outcome and the experienced outcome during and following the exposure—for example, a child who expects to touch a doorknob and get violently ill. Additionally, in the inhibitory learning perspective it is not necessary to provoke anxiety for new learning to occur. Expectancy violation can also be effective if a child can experience a feared situation as humorous or ridiculous. Finally, inhibitory learning encourages SMH professionals to discuss new learning with students after exposures (e.g., "You have touched doorknobs for the last 30 minutes. What have you learned about your fear?"). Because these discussions are associated with greater treatment response among children and adolescents, they are a core component of the inhibitory learning model (Tiwari et al., 2013).

What Is Exposure Therapy?

Exposure therapy is the gold standard, empirically supported treatment for OCD and anxiety disorders, including generalized anxiety disorder, social anxiety, separation anxiety, specific phobia, selective mutism, and panic disorder (Connolly & Bernstein, 2007; Franklin et al., 2015; McGuire et al, 2015; Peterman et al., 2015). Core exposure therapy strategies are applicable across OCD and anxiety disorders, as evidenced by findings that transdiagnostic CBT reduces youth anxiety symptoms across disorders (Bilek & Ehrenreich-May, 2012; Ewing et al., 2015; Zaboski & Storch, 2018). Exposure therapy is an essential component of CBT associated with clinically significant improvements in anxiety symptoms and functional impairment (Ale et al., 2015; Higa-McMillan et al., 2016; Tiwari et al., 2013). The notion that exposure therapy is harmful to children has been repeatedly refuted (e.g., Richard & Gloster, 2007; Schneider et al., 2020; Tryon, 2008; Wang et al., 2017); the treatment is acceptable to parents (Lewin, McGuire, et al., 2014); can be modified to school settings (Zaboski, 2020); and its benefits are well documented (e.g., Franklin et al., 2015; Wang et al., 2017). Adapted approaches to exposure therapy have been found to reduce anxious symptoms in children as young as 4 years of age (Freeman et al., 2014; Lewin, Park, et al., 2014; Rudy et al., 2017) and in children with autism spectrum disorder (Storch et al., 2013; Sukhodolsky et al., 2013; Wood et al., 2019). Exposure therapy can be effective when delivered in a group format (Zaboski et al., 2019), yet in cases of severe social anxiety, trauma histories, or attention-deficit/hyperactivity disorder (ADHD), individual therapy is preferred (Connolly & Bernstein, 2007). In complex cases with multiple comorbidities or more severe symptomotology, it may be indicated to deliver combined psychotherapy and medication intervention (Connolly & Bernstein, 2007).

Exposure Therapy Components
Exposure

Exposure therapy involves in vivo (real life) or imaginal (in one's mind) exposure to distressing stimuli without engaging in avoidance, rituals, or safety behaviors. Exposures include a wide range of therapeutic tasks personalized for the youth's presenting problem. They may consist of brief repetitions of triggering tasks or may be linked to increasingly longer triggering experiences. For example, a student with contamination-focused OCD may be asked to shake hands with people they believe to be contaminated or to maintain physical contact with a "contaminated" doorknob for long periods of time. Critically, after the exposure is completed, the student may not complete safety behaviors or rituals associated with their anxiety, such as handwashing or mental rituals. Types of exposures include in vivo, imaginal, interoceptive, and virtual reality exposure and are discussed in detail in the following paragraphs. Prior to implementing an exposure plan, the therapist should rate the severity of anxiety symptoms using a Subjective Units of Distress Scale (SUDS). This information should be collected before, during, and immediately after the exposure tasks. The SUDS tool typically ranges from 0 (no anxiety) to 10 (panic-attack levels of anxiety). It can be visually depicted for students in several ways, like a thermometer, sliding scale, or smiley faces.

In Vivo Exposure

In vivo exposures occur in real-world situations, whether in therapy sessions or as homework. These exposures can be completely naturalistic, meaning that no one has been informed about the exposure in advance, apart from the client. Alternatively, therapists may give advance notice of the exposure to people involved in the exposure (e.g., parents, teachers) along with instructions for their participation during the task. For example, if an exposure includes answering a challenging question in front of the class, the teacher could be asked in advance to call on that student and report back to the practitioner about the student's behavior during the exposure.

Imaginal Exposure

Imaginal exposures are tasks during which the distressing situation is imagined in detail but not experienced in real life. Imaginal exposures can be helpful for triggers when the fear itself is a thought (like obsessions in OCD), for fears that occur infrequently, or for situations that are impractical or unethical to create in vivo. A child who has a fear of flying, for example, could start by imagining the details of a flight using their five senses (e.g., "Are you in a window or aisle seat?" "What does the plane sound like as you're taking off?"). Next, they could write these details down and repeat them to the therapist in session or to themselves as homework. In later sessions, they may create a worry script, a one-page description of their experience that includes a worst-case scenario coming true (e.g., sitting near someone who is contaminated or a plane crash). The student could then listen to a recording of themselves reading the script or repeatedly read it to themselves as homework.

Interoceptive Exposure

Youth with anxiety are often attuned to bodily signals (shortness of breath, dizziness, nausea, or a racing heartbeat) and develop anxiety in response to them. Interoceptive exposures allow youth to reduce this anxiety. This strategy is particularly useful for children who fear the recurrence of panic attacks because it allows them to experience the bodily sensations of a panic attack without the actual occurrence of one. To induce the physical symptoms, exercises such as shaking one's head back and forth, holding one's breath, breathing through a straw, or running quickly in place may be performed. As always, it is important to get approval from a student's parent, caregiver, or physician to ensure the student does not have an underlying health condition that would respond negatively to these exercises.

Virtual Reality Exposure

Virtual reality exposure is an emerging technology that allows for safe, repeated exposures across a variety of contexts, including exposure to rare or impractical situations (Parsons et al., 2017). Depending on a school's resources, virtual reality exposure could be a promising mode of school-based exposure implementation, although further research is needed to support the efficacy of this strategy among school-aged children (Parsons et al., 2017).

Response Prevention

Response prevention is a core component of exposure therapy in which practitioners minimize avoidant, ritualized, or safety behaviors. While these behaviors may temporarily relieve anxiety at the time of exposure—or, in the case of avoidant behaviors, prevent the exposure altogether—they ultimately sustain or amplify long-term distress. Prior to beginning exposure therapy, the SMH professional should work with the student to determine their avoidance habits, rituals, and safety behaviors. It is critical for parents, and possibly teachers with family permission, to provide information regarding the youth's symptoms to develop an optimal response prevention plan and to provide feedback/support during its implementation. A middle school student may be forthcoming about a ritualized habit of checking and rechecking homework assignments to avoid making a mistake in class. However, an elementary schooler may not realize that he asks the teacher dozens of questions as a safety behavior before an unfamiliar experience, like a field trip. Additionally, parents and teachers often play a central role in these behaviors by accommodating student responses to a trigger. For example, an authority figure may provide reassurance or maintain physical proximity to a student during an anxiety-provoking event. The SMH professional should consult with adults frequently involved in the child's activities to teach them how to reduce their accommodation.

Response prevention is often conducted simultaneously with exposures and, likewise, occurs in a gradual fashion. For the student who repeatedly checks homework assignments, an initial exposure could include completing an assignment and checking all answers only once. After the student performs this task with reduced anxiety, a subsequent exposure could include completing an assignment without checking at all. (Even though checking answers is generally a reasonable study skill, in this case it is important that the student refrain from checking because it interferes with the intervention.) Response prevention must be incorporated into the treatment plan as the experience of a trigger itself is not sufficient to significantly reduce OCD or anxiety symptoms.

Homework

In CBT with exposure therapy, homework is assigned between sessions. This allows for more regular practice of exposures and helps generalize skills outside of the school environment. During sessions, the student and SMH professional conduct exposures and collaborate on additional exposures to practice with a parent or teacher. Depending on the student's progress and motivation, homework may entail repeating the same exposure in session or may involve performance of progressively more distressing tasks. Homework should be tailored to the student's triggers and developmental stage. For example, if the student's main fears are school-specific, homework exposures should be completed at school, whereas a general fear of contamination could be practiced at home or at school. Older students may be able to conduct exposure practice without the aid of a teacher or parent, but younger children often require assistance, so caregivers should be taught how to assist with exposures early in the intervention.

Relapse Prevention

Most students who participate in exposure therapy see a reduction in symptoms (Abramowitz et al., 2005; Wang et al., 2017) that warrant "graduation" from therapy. However, even if anxiety is well managed at termination, future stressors can cause a resurgence of symptoms. Relapse prevention involves planning how to apply therapy skills to future situations to avoid a return of anxiety symptoms.

Psychoeducation about the likelihood of recurring anxiety is an important component of relapse prevention. Through psychoeducation, students learn that their anxiety symptoms may return or may manifest differently and are taught how to utilize their exposure skills to manage future triggers. Students work with counselors to identify triggers, such as starting to ride the bus to school, taking a state achievement test, or transitioning to high school. They also identify likely warning signs of a relapse, such as avoidance of certain activities and excessive reassurance seeking. Students plan their responses to these stressors and create exposure practice tasks for the identified stressors in advance. The student also continues to engage in exposures for the goals that were targeted in therapy, even after therapy has been discontinued.

PARENTAL INVOLVEMENT

As indicated previously, parents strongly influence their child's anxiety, both in symptom severity and response to treatment (Brendel & Maynard, 2014; Lebowitz et al., 2013, 2014). Parents of anxious children often try to make situations less anxiety-provoking by providing verbal reassurance, permitting avoidance, or changing the situation itself (Breinholst et al., 2012; Storch et al., 2007). Accommodating a student's anxiety could involve a parent asking the teacher not to call on their child in class or sitting in on first period every day. Although such responses are understandable, they are unhelpful in the long run as the child does not learn how to cope with their anxiety. Additionally, parents of anxious children frequently model anxious behavior that influences their children's behavior. Due to the impact of parental accommodation and modeled anxious behaviors (Caporino et al., 2012), SMH professionals should include parents in therapy as much as possible, through phone consultation or parent attendance at therapy sessions. Psychoeducation about anxiety disorders and exposure therapy, ways to reduce parental accommodation, and parenting strategies specific to anxious children should be reviewed with parents. A parent handout on exposure therapy can be found in Quick Resource 7.1 in the Appendix.

Developing Fear Hierarchies

A fear hierarchy (or fear ladder) consists of detailed triggers ranked in terms of anticipated distress using the SUDS rating from 0 (no anxiety) to 10 (high anxiety). The initial level consists of a task that evokes minimal distress; incremental steps build to the most distressing challenges. It is important to note that a fear hierarchy is not a list of different anxiety-provoking situations, but an ordered list of gradual steps toward accomplishing a single goal or addressing a specific type of fear (e.g., making mistakes). The same situation (e.g., presenting in front of others) may be modified to create different steps that vary in fear intensity. For example, a student could deliver the same presentation to audiences that are friendly versus critical, familiar versus unknown, and small versus large depending on the student's needs. Steps in the hierarchy should incorporate response prevention targets, such as reducing time spent on the phone with a caregiver each day for a child with separation anxiety. Most students will have multiple hierarchies that address different triggers, although it is generally preferable to combine them into a comprehensive hierarchy for the sake of parsimony and to convey that exposure therapy is transdiagnostic. To do this, a student with separation anxiety and specific phobia (fear of the dark and burglars) could work through a single hierarchy with the goal of sleeping independently without a night light and without repeatedly checking windows and locks. Refer to Quick Resource 7.2 in the Appendix for examples of fear hierarchies.

Students should be involved in creating their fear hierarchy. While the SMH professional, parent, or teacher may have a good understanding of the child's anxiety or fear, the student often best understands how different variables impact their anxiety. For example, some students with OCD who struggle with contamination fears may find it more difficult to eat lunch without first washing their hands for an extended period of time, while others may find it more difficult to eat lunch without first sanitizing their utensils. Incorporating the student's ideas into the hierarchy can increase their engagement in the therapeutic process.

Students may be more motivated to address some fears than others; for example, if they wish to attend sleepovers, they may be more willing to address separation anxiety fears first. Reinforcement of "brave" behaviors through praise or rewards is encouraged to build student engagement. SMH professionals can create a menu of rewards and determine which exposures the student will complete to earn each reward. Rewards should be tailored to the student's developmental stage and the difficulty of their therapeutic goals. For example, stickers and snacks may motivate younger students, whereas older students may choose screen time or a small purchase. Teachers and parents are useful partners in delivering rewards and should be consulted for no-cost reinforcers, such as being the line leader or picking what the family has for dinner. Finally, creating fear hierarchies to guide exposure practice is a skill that students can learn and practice on their own.

Students can assist in creating a fear hierarchy in several different ways. If the student has been introduced to a system to rate anxiety-provoking situations (e.g., SUDS), then the SMH professional can use that system to instruct students to add to the hierarchy. Students who struggle with a SUDS system can be prompted to rate situations in comparison to each other to form the hierarchy (e.g., "Would raising your hand be easier or harder than walking to your teacher's desk?"). Note that the examples provided in Quick Resource 7.2 will vary from student to student.

Treatment Progression

Treatment progression should be individualized to each student. The primary factor to consider is the severity of a student's anxiety, which will inform hierarchy development, when to move on to the next exposure, and when the intervention is finished. There is no set number of levels in a fear hierarchy. Triggers that are more anxiety-provoking may require additional steps. If there is a large gap between steps in the fear hierarchy (e.g., if one is rated 3/10 and the next is rated 7/10), intermediate steps should be created. For example, a child who experiences anxiety asking for help may rate asking a peer to borrow a pencil as 3/10 and asking a teacher for help with a homework assignment as 7/10. In this case, intermediate steps should be created between these exposure challenges (e.g., asking the teacher for a pencil, asking the teacher to use the restroom, asking a peer for help with an assignment). Fear hierarchies should be fluid and adaptable, and SMH professionals should be prepared to add or eliminate challenges as needed.

Traditional exposure practice begins at the first level of the fear hierarchy and moves up to each subsequent level during intervention. In the habituation or emotional processing models, the length of time spent on each level will depend on the time it takes a student's anxiety to decrease. However, the inhibitory learning model de-emphasizes this stepwise approach, suggesting that variability in the order, stimuli, and duration of exposures maximizes the intervention effects (Craske et al., 2014). Practitioners should balance the need for variable difficulty with the student's ability to tolerate more difficult exposures. As a student progresses through the hierarchy, subsequent exposures may be eliminated or modified as progress generalizes. Daily practice should be assigned for about 30 to 60 minutes, but while students should be challenged during exposure practice, they should never be overwhelmed.

Exposure-based interventions do not progress with the goal of eliminating anxiety completely; rather, the interventions reduce excessive anxiety, allow students to tolerate discomfort, and enable clients to participate in normative activities even if they provoke anxiety. Specific behavioral goals, which guide the creation of fear hierarchies, should be established at the beginning of therapy. Students often benefit from creating a "bonus" step in the fear hierarchy that is even more anxiety-provoking than the ultimate goal, since this helps them to achieve new learning and gain confidence. For example, if a student wants to present in front of the class, an extra "bonus" step may be a presentation in front of an even larger group. Other strategies to strengthen intervention outcomes include deepened extinction and exposure in multiple contexts (Craske et al., 2014). Deepened extinction works by amplifying expectancy violation during an exposure. For example, a student with contamination fears may ordinarily complete two exposures: (1) touching the door handle to the cafeteria without washing their hands afterward and (2) eating at the cafeteria table without wiping it down. The deepened extinction method would involve completing both tasks within the same exercise: touching a cafeteria doorknob, then immediately sitting down at an unwiped table to eat lunch. Conducting exposures in multiple contexts can help to generalize the effects of exposure and to prevent relapses. In the school setting, variations in context could include class period, location in the school building, number of people present, and being around only adults or only students.

Additionally, intervention is never "finished." Although the child may not be engaging in active exposure practice, they should still be engaged in the situations on a regular basis as part of typical school activities. For example, if a student with performance anxiety succeeded in performing a practiced speech, they could continue to engage in class-based participation and presentations after their goal is achieved. Many students will benefit from booster exposure practices to maintain their engagement in anxiety-provoking activities, to address new fears that emerged, and to motivate further practice.

COGNITIVE RESTRUCTURING WITH EXPOSURE

The goal of cognitive restructuring, as explained in Chapter 6, is to replace a maladaptive thought with a thought based on reason and evidence. Cognitive restructuring paired with exposure therapy can help students successfully complete exposures. However, exposure therapy should remain the primary approach for anxiety reduction in CBT because it is the component of CBT that leads to the greatest anxiety symptom reduction (e.g., Vande Voort et al., 2010).

Cognitive Skills During Exposure Therapy

When cognitive restructuring is integrated with exposure therapy, SMH professionals should remind students about the triadic relationship between thoughts, feelings, and behaviors that they learned about through psychoeducation. They can connect how students' cognitions influence their behavior and feelings (physical and emotional) during exposures. They can also explore how engagement in exposure alters their cognitions and feelings.

To challenge worried thoughts, the SMH provider works through a series of questions with the student to explore their expectations for the exposure. The following questions prompt the student to find evidence for and against a worried thought:

- How likely is it?
- What would a friend predict would happen?
- What has happened before?
- What could be another explanation?
- What evidence do you have for and against your prediction?
- From a scale of 0 (no anxiety) to 10 (maximum anxiety), how worried are you about this task?

Once a student has practiced cognitive restructuring several times, they can create a "cheat sheet" of questions and phrases they can refer to that they find helpful in reducing their anxiety. Parents and teachers involved in the intervention can prompt students to use it when they observe or anticipate anxious behavior.

During an exposure, students may use the cognitive strategy of self-statements like "I can do hard things" or "I am brave" to cope with anxious feelings. The statements can also be provided by the SMH provider, teachers, and parents as reinforcement (e.g., "You are so brave!"). Self-statements can serve as a modified strategy for younger children or children with comorbid disabilities for whom cognitive restructuring is too abstract or demanding. Practitioners are reminded that these statements differ from statements that accommodate anxiety. For instance, it is appropriate to praise a child for completing an exposure to touch a doorknob ("You can do it!"), but be wary of statements that include reassurance such as, "You can do it! You'll be OK!" This is because the student should learn *through the exposure* that they will be OK, not through the practitioner's reassurance.

When to Use Cognitive Restructuring with Exposure Therapy

DEVELOPMENTAL AND DISABILITY CONSIDERATIONS

Young students may not have the cognitive or linguistic skills required for cognitive restructuring. Additionally, students with intellectual or developmental disabilities may struggle to engage in cognitive restructuring due to deficits in social perspective-taking, communication skills, or intellectual ability (Wood et al., 2009). Although cognitive restructuring may not be an appropriate strategy for some young students and students with disabilities, exposure therapy can be conducted successfully in these populations without the use of cognitive strategies (Rudy et al., 2017; Sukhodolsky et al., 2013; Wood et al., 2009).

TIME CONSIDERATIONS

In the school setting, time is a precious resource, and SMH professionals may be hard pressed to find a time to schedule therapy sessions. Students miss less academic content when therapy is brief and effective at meeting their goals. When students start exposures earlier in therapy rather than spending multiple sessions on psychoeducation and cognitive skills, they achieve the same level of symptom reduction but experience remission more quickly (Gryczkowski et al., 2013; Vande Voort et al., 2010). Therefore, practitioners should balance the benefits of cognitive restructuring with the time it takes *away* from exposures.

INHIBITORY LEARNING PERSPECTIVE ON COGNITIVE RESTRUCTURING

Within inhibitory learning, the greatest symptom reduction occurs when expectations are violated through exposure. Proponents claim that because certain cognitive behavioral strategies (e.g., cognitive restructuring, coping) reduce the intensity of a feared outcome, they reduce the effectiveness of exposures (Craske et al., 2014). Craske et al. recommended that rather than utilizing cognitive skills before or during exposures, cognitive skills should be used after exposure to debrief about expected outcomes, experienced outcomes, and expectancy violation. For example, a student with a specific phobia of school mascots could practice watching a pep rally from the hallway of the gym. Afterward, she could discuss what she feared would happen, what she experienced, and the discrepancy between the two outcomes. Professionals should monitor if youth use cognitive restructuring as a safety behavior, distraction, or a stalling technique (Peterman et al., 2015). The student who fears mascots might repeat to herself "mascots never hurt anyone" over and over to the point that the cognitive strategy is a ritual or safety behavior that only temporarily relieves anxiety. As a guideline, Peterman et al. suggest that cognitive restructuring should not be used when it promotes avoidance.

In summary, the potential benefits of cognitive strategies must be balanced with possible costs (less efficient interventions, decreasing expectancy violation, and potentially introducing safety behaviors). Cognitive strategies can build confidence and engagement, especially when baseline anxiety levels are high. Students may also find that cognitive restructuring is a helpful tool for novel anxiety-provoking situations when exposures are less practical.

EXPOSURE THERAPY AND TRAUMA

Exposure to traumatic events during childhood and adolescence is not uncommon, with approximately two-thirds of students experiencing at least one adverse event during their school-aged years (Gonzalez et al., 2016; Jaycox et al., 2002). It is not surprising, then, that best practices for school-based, trauma-informed screening, assessment, and intervention practices have been developed and given thoughtful discussion (Chafouleas et al., 2016; Eklund et al., 2018). School-based mental health services offer increased access to treatment, overcoming many barriers to treatment access (e.g., lack of transportation, having to locate childcare for siblings, insufficient time; McKay & Bannon, 2004). This is particularly relevant for the delivery of trauma-focused treatments, with only 15% of youth completing treatment in community-based clinics and 91% completing trauma treatment in schools (Jaycox et al., 2010). With schools as integral providers of trauma-focused care, it is important that SMH professionals are familiar with the core components of trauma-focused therapy and implications for school-based implementation. Trauma-focused cognitive behavior therapy (TF-CBT; Cohen et al., 2017) is a well-established, evidence-based practice for youth exposed to traumatic events (Silverman et al., 2008). This section focuses on the exposure components of TF-CBT, including trauma narratives and in vivo exposures.

Trauma Narratives

A trauma narrative is the story of a student's traumatic event written in detail. The process of developing a trauma narrative is considered a core component for the treatment of posttraumatic stress. Both constructing the narrative and processing the narrative help to modify maladaptive fears associated with the traumatic event (Amaya-Jackson & DeRosa, 2007; Rauch & Foa, 2006). Developing and sharing the narrative are considered exposure techniques that facilitate desensitization to reminders of the trauma, reduce avoidance behaviors, and decrease physiological arousal. As students are repeatedly exposed to their narrative through writing it and sharing it with others, they learn to disconnect the thoughts and reminders of the trauma from the negative emotions linked to it, including terror, anxiety, fear, hopelessness, anger, or shame.

Exposure to the narrative is gradual, progressing according to the student's level of anxiety and avoidance. Students with high anxiety and avoidance may start with small tasks such as giving the narrative a title or table of contents, setting a timer to show how much time will be spent on it within session, or writing a neutral narrative (Cohen et al., 2017). During trauma narration, the SMH professional may act as the student's scribe. At the end of each section, the student is asked to read what has been written before moving to the next section. If there are reading difficulties or reticence for reading content aloud, the SMH professional can read sections to the student. As each section is constructed and reviewed, the SMH professional should assess for emotional distress (e.g., SUDS) and initiate relaxation techniques as indicated. (Note that practitioners should *not* generally initiate relaxation strategies for exposures that do not involve trauma.) Once regulated, the SMH professional should praise the student and return to the narrative rather than discontinue it, as this may encourage avoidance. The repetition of content promotes reduction in emotional distress and physiological reactivity. After the narrative is completed, the SMH professional should ask the student to identify the worst moments and the thoughts, feelings, and physical sensations related to them. These moments will be targeted in subsequent sessions through cognitive processing (discussed next).

Cognitive Processing of the Trauma Narrative

Cognitive processing is the act of challenging maladaptive trauma-related cognitions. Maladaptive cognitions are often inaccurate (e.g., "I should have known he would assault me"; it is my fault my mom died") or unhelpful (e.g., "I can't trust men because they will hurt me"). Cognitive processing includes strategies such as progressive logical questioning and the "responsibility pie."

Progressive logical questioning is used first. In this exercise, the student is presented with a cognitive behavioral triangle featuring the maladaptive thought and works toward replacing the thought with a more helpful or accurate thought. The student may have made active or passive decisions that increased vulnerability to the trauma. As such, a practitioner may need to help them distinguish between learning from mistakes (e.g., "I drank too much and regret that") and being responsible for what happened (e.g., "I am not responsible for being assaulted").

The responsibility pie activity can be used to demonstrate the differences between responsibility and regret and the role each party may have had in the event. During this activity, the client is asked to divide the responsibility for the event among everyone involved. Progressive logical questioning can be used to help the child allocate responsibility while acknowledging any regret they may have about their decisions (Cohen et al., 2017).

Parent Involvement in the Trauma Narrative

Parent involvement in TF-CBT improves child outcomes (Cohen et al., 2017; Deblinger et al., 1996), and SMH professionals are strongly encouraged to engage the student's parent or caregiver in the intervention. Students typically work on narrative development while the SMH professional meets with the parent concurrently. During parent meetings, the SMH professional should conduct a readiness assessment to determine the parent's willingness to support the child; ability to manage their own distress (e.g., tearful, angry, vengeful); specific anxieties about discussing the trauma; and willingness to engage in conjoint sessions with the student (see Cohen & Mannarino, 1996, 1998, 2000). Children with parents who present with avoidance and shame tend to have poorer prognoses over time (Yasinski et al., 2016) and may express more concern about sharing the narrative with them. (Beliefs that parents will be upset or mad are common.) Consequently, practitioners should discuss with clients the level of detail that they are comfortable sharing as well as the conditions under which sharing will stop (e.g., parent becomes too upset).

After discussing the parameters of the conjoint session, the primary goals are for the parent to model adaptive behaviors when hearing about the trauma, for the child to experience reduced anxiety, and for the dyad to feel empowered to have healthy discussions about the trauma (Cohen et al., 2017).

Notably, there may be situations where the parent cannot or will not participate in treatment (e.g., the parent was the perpetrator of the child's trauma, the child is in a foster home, the parents are deceased) and the narrative cannot be shared. In these cases, it may be helpful for SMH professionals to collaborate with trusted adults in the child's life (e.g., foster parents, direct care providers in a group home). When adult participation is not possible, SMH professionals should note that youth can still experience symptom improvement (Cohen et al., 2017).

In Vivo Exposure

After completing the trauma narrative and cognitive processing, many youth experience reductions in anxiety (Deblinger et al., 2015). In these cases, in vivo exposure may not be needed. Some youth develop overgeneralized fears of innocuous stimuli (e.g., the bedroom when an assault happened) or have trauma cues that are associated with underlying themes of their trauma (e.g., everyday relationships triggering themes of betrayal; Cohen et al., 2012; Saxe et al., 2007) and may benefit from in vivo exposure to these stimuli. Often children and youth believe that avoidance will help them master events that led to past traumas and prevent future ones. Ongoing assessment of trauma themes and associated distress can help SMH professionals know when in vivo exposures may be indicated. The exposures may be performed before, during, or after narrative development.

Ideally, the SMH professional will include the parent during in vivo exposure planning. Collaboratively, a fear hierarchy is developed, and rewards are designated for completion of the in vivo exposure activities. Praise should be provided for approach behaviors (e.g., taking steps toward performing an exposure) as well as achieving hierarchy items. As in exposure therapy for anxiety, exposure homework between sessions is often assigned, and the practitioner should assess homework progress and help to overcome any obstacles. For example, in vivo exposure would be appropriate for a student who has an ongoing fear of showering at home due to a traumatic event that occurred in a gym restroom at school. Early steps of a hierarchy for this student could include standing in the bathroom alone at home and running the shower water but not getting in. As in exposure therapy for anxiety disorders, in vivo exposure can include a fading of safety behaviors, such as starting with a parent present and then asking the parent to be farther and farther away from the shower stall for subsequent exposures.

In trauma-focused work, it is particularly important for SMH professionals to assess whether fears related to trauma cues are innocuous or reality-based. In some cases, a student's anxiety may function to keep them safe. For example, if a child is at risk of ongoing abuse when going to visit a family member who has abused them in the past, in vivo activities should *not* focus on desensitizing anxiety to these cues. Reality-based safety concerns should result in safety planning and are not appropriate targets for in vivo exposures (Cohen et al., 2017; Fitzgerald & Cohen, 2012). Safety planning for students who are exposed to ongoing violence or trauma in their community could include teaching them to recognize and be aware of antecedents to violence so that they can remove themselves from imminent danger.

Complex Trauma

For students with complex trauma, or an experience of multiple traumatic events, it may be difficult to isolate a specific trauma for narrative construction due to fragmentation and the non-linear nature of complex trauma memories. The SMH professional should work collaboratively with the student to discover cross-cutting trauma-related themes as the focus of treatment (e.g., self-blame, lack of trust, being damaged; Cohen et al., 2017) rather than a discrete event or experience. Together, the dyad reviews narrative content for core trauma themes, with the SMH professional helping the student connect themes to current maladaptive cognitions (Cohen et al., 2012).

TF-CBT Implementation Considerations

Several student and clinician behaviors can influence the success of TF-CBT. Practitioners should note any avoidance (e.g., refusing to participate in session activities, insisting that avoidance is an effective way of coping), an indicator of intervention dropout (Yasinski et al., 2018). Providers should also monitor their own actions to prevent reinforcement of avoidance behaviors (e.g., ending a session prematurely with a student who is not engaged). Generally, an empathic and supportive approach is critical with trauma-exposed students, given potentially high levels of interpersonal mistrust. Strategies such as allocating time for positive activities at the end of session (e.g., games, discussion of personal interests) and reinforcing participation through praise and rewards can promote continued engagement (Fitzgerald & Cohen, 2012).

Implications for TF-CBT in School Settings

Integrating school mental health programming into a larger model (e.g., multi-tiered systems of support [MTSS]) or other systems of support can enhance service delivery (Weist et al., 2018). For example, an MTSS team could monitor TF-CBT effectiveness through a Tier 2 behavior support like Check In/Check Out (CICO; Crone et al., 2010). Consider a student with a trauma history (e.g., being bullied). If they have difficulty engaging in routine school activities, CICO could help prompt them to engage in basic breathing or relaxation strategies to meet Tier 1 behavior expectations. With these strategies designated as target behaviors, teachers have increased awareness that these are skills in development and may be willing to promote their generalization to the classroom (Weist et al., 2018).

Another school-specific consideration relates to consent. Practitioners should explain the purpose and limits of information sharing (e.g., observing the student in class, offering the teacher strategies to address student distress) and how these strategies can expedite recovery. In the absence of this information, students and parents may erroneously believe that the teachers will receive detailed information about the family's mental health history or about the trauma narrative and be reluctant to participate.

Lastly, school personnel may be concerned that TF-CBT interferes with academic instruction. There may be some truth to this. Students may be unable to engage in intense learning activities after narrative development or a processing session if their focus is still on the narrative (Fitzgerald & Cohen, 2012). However, practitioners can alleviate this problem by allocating time immediately after the session to help the student relax before returning to the classroom. For example, clients might engage in less anxiety-provoking activities, like coloring, playing games, or watching videos before leaving the session.

Stepped-Care Models for School-Based TF-CBT

Stepped-care TF-CBT (SC-TF-CBT; Salloum, Robst, et al., 2014) is a two-step TF-CBT adaptation designed as an accessible and cost-effective front-line treatment for trauma-exposed youth. On average, three-quarters of school counselors have more than 250 students on their caseloads (Shi & Brown, 2020), with an average of 83 of these students requiring behavioral health treatment (Christian & Brown, 2018), which makes it difficult to see every student for weekly sessions. Prior to individual therapy, SC-TF-CBT begins with a parent-led, therapist-assisted treatment approach (Step 1) that is primarily conducted at home with an intervention workbook. To facilitate this, professionals meet with parents for 60 minutes three times over the course of several weeks. Phone consultations with the SMH provider are also included. Following Step 1, children in need of further treatment proceed to a full course of TF-CBT (see Salloum, Scheeringa, et al., 2014, for more information on SC-TF-CBT). Further investigation in clinical trials using larger samples is needed to identify characteristics of responders/non-responders to Step 1 and to test treatment moderators for this modality. Findings could guide SMH professionals on which cases would be ideal for SC-TF-CBT and how to identify families who would be a best fit for this intervention.

EXPOSURE THERAPY CASE REPORT

This section provides a sample case of school-based exposure therapy for a 10-year-old girl, Michelle, with social anxiety. Michelle was referred by her 5th-grade teacher for general education counseling. She noticed that Michelle avoided talking to other students during group work and recess, became distressed when asked to answer a question or read aloud in class, and required assistance ordering her food in the cafeteria line. Even when she did high-quality work, Michelle refused to let the teacher share it with the class or post it on the wall. When the school psychologist, Ms. Smith, called Michelle's parents to receive consent for counseling, Michelle's parents noted that her anxiety got in the way of her attending social and extracurricular activities. She also tried to stay home on days when there was a performance or class party.

Ms. Smith invited Michelle's parents to attend the first counseling session, and her mother attended. This session was devoted to gathering more information about Michelle's fears and the family's responses to them, as well as providing psychoeducation about exposure therapy for anxiety. It was determined that Michelle's main fears included being humiliated and socially rejected by her peers. When Michelle tried to avoid a social encounter, her parents repeatedly reassured her that "everything will be OK," and they brainstormed ways to make the event less scary, like attending it with her. If her anxiety still reached unacceptably high levels, her parents let her skip the event entirely. Ms. Smith explained how avoidance maintains anxiety long-term, even if it relieves it in the moment, and how exposure to distressing situations reduces anxiety. She connected how both Michelle's avoidance and her parents' accommodation (e.g., providing excessive reassurance, making events less anxiety-provoking, allowing her to skip events) maintained her anxiety. She explained how Michelle's role in counseling was to participate in exposures, both in and outside of sessions, and her parents' role was to support exposure practice and reduce accommodation. Ms. Smith and Michelle collaborated on the first fear hierarchy, and Ms. Smith explained how to practice exposures, complete a homework log, and provide SUDS ratings. They created a rewards menu together with small rewards for exposure tasks and a larger reward for intervention completion.

In the subsequent sessions, Ms. Smith met with Michelle individually. During each session, they completed in vivo exposures and planned exposures for homework. The goal of Michelle's first hierarchy was to hold conversations with peers at recess. The hierarchy started with standing close to familiar classmates and progressed to saying hello to familiar classmates and ultimately holding back-and-forth conversations with less familiar peers. The sessions were scheduled to overlap with recess, so Michelle could complete exposures and then debrief with Ms. Smith. Before, during, and after exposures, Michelle provided SUDS ratings, and an exposure continued until her rating reduced by about half. After the exposures, they discussed how Michelle's feared outcome compared to the experienced outcome. For homework, Michelle was assigned similar exposures to practice at her extracurricular activities (e.g., Girl Scouts, dance).

As Michelle familiarized herself with CBT, her therapist started a second hierarchy to address her fear of answering questions in class and worked with Michelle's teacher to implement it. As an early step, the teacher confirmed with Michelle privately that her work was correct before asking her to answer a question that required a single-word response (e.g., true or false). Later steps included providing brief answers to simple questions and answering more challenging questions without checking her work. The reduction of work checking was an example of response prevention through the fading of safety behaviors. Michelle's final exposure was to provide an incorrect answer in front of the class. Although this task made her feel uncomfortable, she discussed with Ms. Smith afterward how her anxious feelings only lasted a few minutes, and no one laughed at her as she feared they would. Through each task on the hierarchy, Michelle received praise for her brave behavior from Ms. Smith, her teacher, and her parents. She also received some small rewards such as extra computer time and special snacks.

Once Michelle could engage in several social situations with manageable anxiety, Ms. Smith spoke with the family about terminating counseling. Her parents both attended the final session on relapse prevention. Together, they celebrated Michelle's progress and collaborated on her final reward. Ms. Smith reviewed the concepts and strategies that Michelle had learned so that the family could apply them to manage future anxiety symptoms. They discussed potential future stressors and how the strategies could be applied in those situations. For example, anticipating Michelle's transition to middle school next year, she planned to practice talking to unfamiliar peers in the weeks preceding the start of school. Ms. Smith also reviewed ways that Michelle's parents could reduce accommodations by requiring her to attend new social events without giving excessive reassurance. Finally, they talked about the possibility of pursuing counseling services at the new school should symptoms return or intensify.

CHAPTER DISCUSSION QUESTIONS

1. Describe the similarities and differences between the proposed mechanisms of change across the theories of cognitive behavioral therapy with exposure.

2. In what situations (populations, diagnoses, impairment, etc.) is CBT with exposure indicated as an appropriate treatment?
3. What are the different types of exposures, and in what situations are they most beneficial?
4. What is relapse prevention and why is it useful?
5. How are schools uniquely suited to provide trauma-focused CBT? On the other hand, in what situations would administrators, teachers, or parents be reluctant to support the delivery of TF-CBT in the schools?
6. What types of exposure strategies are used in TF-CBT? How is the use of exposure in TF-CBT similar to and different from the use of exposure in non–trauma-exposed students?
7. A 2nd-grader has separation anxiety. Each morning he cries and pleads with his mother in the parking lot for an hour to not make him go to school. Eventually, she gets him in the building after the school counselor meets them at the car and sits with him for most of his first period. Using exposure and response prevention, what should the counselor do to improve this student's daily functioning?

REFERENCES

Abramowitz, J. S., Whiteside, S. P., & Deacon, B. J. (2005). The effectiveness of treatment for pediatric obsessive-compulsive disorder: A meta-analysis. *Behavior Therapy*, 36(1), 55–63. https://doi.org/10.1016/S0005-7894(05)80054-1

Ale, C. M., McCarthy, D. M., Rothschild, L. M., & Whiteside, S. P. (2015). Components of cognitive behavioral therapy related to outcome in childhood anxiety disorders. *Clinical Child and Family Psychology Review*, 18(3), 240–251. https://doi.org/10.1007/s10567-015-0184-8

Amaya-Jackson, L., & DeRosa, R. (2007). Treatment considerations for clinicians in applying evidence-based practice to complex presentations of child trauma. *Journal of Traumatic Stress*, 20, 379–390. https://doi.org/10.1002/jts.20266

Benito, K. G., & Walther, M. (2015). Therapeutic process during exposure: Habituation model. *Journal of Obsessive-Compulsive and Related Disorders*, 6, 147–157. https://doi.org/10.1016/j.jocrd.2015.01.006

Bergez, K. C., Ramirez, A. C., Grebe, S. C., Perez, M. I., Viana, A. G., Storch, E. A., & Schneider, S. C. (2020). Efficacy of exposure-based cognitive behavioral therapy for youth anxiety and obsessive-compulsive disorder. In T. S. Peris, E. A. Storch, & J. F. McGuire (Eds.), *Exposure therapy for children with anxiety and OCD* (pp. 21–37). Academic Press.

Bilek, E. L., & Ehrenreich-May, J. (2012). An open trial investigation of a transdiagnostic group treatment for children with anxiety and depressive symptoms. *Behavior Therapy*, 43(4), 887–897. https://doi.org/10.1016/j.beth.2012.04.007Breinholst, S., Esbjorn, B. H., Reinholdt-Dunne, M. L., & Stallard, P. (2012). CBT for the treatment of child anxiety disorders: A review of why parental involvement has not enhanced outcomes. *Journal of Anxiety Disorders*, 26(3), 416–424. https://doi.org/10.1016/j.janxdis.2011.12.014

Brendel, K. E., & Maynard, B. R. (2014). Child–parent interventions for childhood anxiety disorders: A systematic review and meta-analysis. *Research on Social Work Practice, 24*(3), 287–295. https://doi.org/10.1177/1049731513503713

Caporino, N. E., Morgan, J., Beckstead, J., Phares, V., Murphy, T. K., & Storch, E. A. (2012). A structural equation analysis of family accommodation in pediatric obsessive-compulsive disorder. *Journal of Abnormal Child Psychology, 40*(1), 133–143. https://doi.org/10.1007/s10802-011-9549-8

Chafouleas, S. M., Johnson, A. H., Overstreet, S., & Santos, N. M. (2016). Toward a blueprint for trauma-informed service delivery in schools. *School Mental Health, 8,* 144–162. https://doi.org/10.1007/s12310-015-9166-8

Christian, D. D., & Brown, C. L. (2018). Recommendations for the role and responsibilities of school-based mental health counselors. *Journal of School-Based Counseling Policy and Evaluation, 1,* 26–39. https://doi.org/10.25774/nmfk-y245

Cohen, J. A., & Mannarino, A. P. (1996). A treatment outcome study for sexually abused preschool children: Initial findings. *Journal of the American Academy of Child and Adolescent Psychiatry, 35*(1), 42–50. https://doi.org/10.1097/00004583-199601000-00011

Cohen, J. A., & Mannarino, A. P. (1998). Interventions for sexually abused children: Initial treatment outcome findings. *Child Maltreatment, 5*(1), 17–26. https://doi.org/10.1177/1077559598003001002

Cohen, J. A., & Mannarino, A. P. (2000). Predictors of treatment outcome in sexually abused children. *Child Abuse & Neglect, 24*(7), 983–994. https://doi.org/10.1016/s0145-2134(00)00153-8

Cohen, J. A., Mannarino, A. P., & Deblinger, E. (2017). *Treating trauma and traumatic grief in children and adolescents* (2nd ed.). Guilford Press. https://doi.org/10.1016/j.chiabu.2012.03.007

Cohen, J. A., Mannarino, A. P., Kliethermes, M., & Murray, L. A. (2012). Trauma-focused CBT for youth with complex trauma. *Child Abuse & Neglect, 36,* 528–541.

Connolly, S. D., & Bernstein, G. A. (2007). Practice parameter for the assessment and treatment of children and adolescents with anxiety disorders. *Journal of the American Academy of Child & Adolescent Psychiatry, 46*(2), 267–283. https://doi.org/10.1097/01.chi.0000246070.23695.06

Craske, M. G., Kircanski, K., Zelikowsky, M., Mystkowski, J., Chowdhury, N., & Baker, A. (2008). Optimizing inhibitory learning during exposure therapy. *Behaviour Research and Therapy, 46*(1), 5–27. https://doi.org/10.1016/j.brat.2007.10.003

Craske, M. G., Treanor, M., Conway, C. C., Zbozinek, T., & Vervliet, B. (2014). Maximizing exposure therapy: An inhibitory learning approach. *Behaviour Research and Therapy, 58,* 10–23. https://doi.org/10.1016/j.brat.2014.04.006

Crone, D. A., Hawken, L. S., & Horner, R. H. (2010). *Responding to problem behavior in schools: The behavior education program.* Guilford Press.

Dawson, R., & McMurray, N. (1978). Desensitization without hierarchical presentation and concomitant relaxation. *Australian Journal of Psychology, 30*(2), 119–132.

Deblinger, E., Lippmann, J., & Steer, R. (1996). Sexually abused children suffering posttraumatic stress symptoms: Initial treatment outcome findings. *Child Maltreatment, 1*(4), 310–321. https://doi.org/10.1177/1077559596001004003

Deblinger, E., Mannarino, A. P., Cohen, J. A. (Eds.), Runyon, M. K., & Heflin, A. H. (Collaborators). (2015). *Child sexual abuse: A primer for treating children, adolescents, and their nonoffending parents* (2nd ed.). Oxford University Press.

Eklund, K., Rossen, E., Koriakin, T., Chafouleas, S. M., & Resnick, C. (2018). A systematic review of trauma screening measures for children and adolescents. *School Psychology Quarterly*, *33*(1), 30–43. https://doi.org/10.1037/spq0000244

Ewing, D. L., Monsen, J. J., Thompson, E. J., Cartwright-Hatton, S., & Field, A. (2015). A meta-analysis of transdiagnostic cognitive behavioural therapy in the treatment of child and young person anxiety disorders. *Behavioural and Cognitive Psychotherapy*, *43*(5), 562–577. https://doi.org/10.1017/S1352465813001094

Fitzgerald, M. M., & Cohen, J. A. (2012) Trauma-focused cognitive behavior therapy for school psychologists. *Journal of Applied School Psychology*, *28*(3), 294–315. https://doi.org/10.1080/15377903.2012.696037

Foa, E. B., & Kozak, M. J. (1986). Emotional processing of fear: Exposure to corrective information. *Psychological Bulletin*, *99*(1), 20–35. https://doi.org/10.1037/0033-2909.99.1.20

Foa, E. B., & McLean, C. P. (2016). The efficacy of exposure therapy for anxiety-related disorders and its underlying mechanisms: The case of OCD and PTSD. *Annual Review of Clinical Psychology*, *12*, 1–28. https://doi.org/10.1146/annurev-clinpsy-021815-093533

Franklin, M. E., Kratz, H. E., Freeman, J. B., Ivarsson, T., Heyman, I., Sookman, D., McKay, D., Storch, E. A., March, J., & Accreditation Task Force of the Canadian Institute for Obsessive Compulsive Disorders. (2015). Cognitive-behavioral therapy for pediatric obsessive-compulsive disorder: Empirical review and clinical recommendations. *Psychiatry Research*, *227*(1), 78–92. https://doi.org/10.1016/j.psychres.2015.02.009

Freeman, J., Sapyta, J., Garcia, A., Compton, S., Khanna, M., Flessner, C., FitzGerald, D., Mauro, C., Dingfelder, R., Benito, K., Harrison, J., Curry, J., Foa, E., March, J., Moore, P., & Franklin, M. (2014). Family-based treatment of early childhood obsessive-compulsive disorder: The pediatric obsessive-compulsive disorder treatment study for young children (POTS Jr)—a randomized clinical trial. *JAMA Psychiatry*, *71*(6), 689–698. https://doi.org/10.1001/jamapsychiatry.2014.170

Gillan, P., & Rachman, S. (1974). An experimental investigation of desensitization in phobic patients. *British Journal of Psychiatry*, *124*(581), 392–401. https://doi.org/10.1192/bjp.124.4.392

Gonzalez, A., Monzon, N., Solis, D., Jaycox, L., & Langley, A. K., (2016). Trauma exposure in elementary school children: Description of screening procedures, level of exposure, and stress symptoms. *School Mental Health*, *8*, 77–88. https://doi.org/10.1007/s12310-015-9167-7

Gryczkowski, M. R., Tiede, M. S., Dammann, J. E., Brown Jacobsen, A., Hale, L. R., & Whiteside, S. P. (2013). The timing of exposure in clinic-based treatment for childhood anxiety disorders. *Behavior Modification*, *37*(1), 113–127. https://doi.org/10.1177/0145445513482394

Hezel, D. M., & Simpson, H. B. (2019). Exposure and response prevention for obsessive-compulsive disorder: A review and new directions. *Indian Journal of Psychiatry*, *61*, 85–92. https://doi.org/10.4103/psychiatry.IndianJPsychiatry_516_18

Higa-McMillan, C. K., Francis, S. E., Rith-Najarian, L., & Chorpita, B. F. (2016). Evidence base update: 50 years of research on treatment for child and adolescent anxiety. *Journal of Clinical Child & Adolescent Psychology*, *45*(2), 91–113. https://doi.org/10.1080/15374416.2015.1046177

Jaycox, L. H., Cohen, J. A., Mannarino, A. P., Walker, D. W., Langley, A. K., Gegenheimer, K. L., Scott, M., & Schonlau, M. (2010). Children's mental health care following Hurricane Katrina: A field trial of trauma-focused psychotherapies. *Journal of Traumatic Stress, 23*(2), 223–231. https://doi.org/10.1002/jts.20518

Jaycox, L. H., Stein, B. D., Kataoka, S. H., Wong, M., Fink, A., Escudero, P., & Zaragoza, C. (2002). Violence exposure, posttraumatic stress disorder, and depressive symptoms among recent immigrant school children. *Journal of the American Academy of Child and Adolescent Psychiatry, 41*, 1104–1110. https://doi.org/10.1097/00004583-200209000-00011

Johnco, C., McGuire, J. F., Roper, T., & Storch, E. A. (2020). A meta-analysis of dropout rates from exposure with response prevention and pharmacological treatment for youth with obsessive compulsive disorder. *Depression and Anxiety, 37*(5), 407–417. https://doi.org/10.1002/da.22978

Lader, M. H., & Wing, L (1966). *Physiological measures, sedative drugs and morbid anxiety*. Oxford University Press.

Lang, P. J., & Lazovik, A. D. (1963). Experimental desensitization of a phobia. *Journal of Abnormal and Social Psychology, 66*, 519–525. https://doi.org/10.1037/h0039828

Lebowitz, E. R., Omer, H., Hermes, H., & Scahill, L. (2014). Parent training for childhood anxiety disorders: The SPACE program. *Cognitive and Behavioral Practice, 21*(4), 456–469. https://doi.org/10.1016/j.cbpra.2013.10.004

Lebowitz, E. R., Woolston, J., Bar-Haim, Y., Calvocoressi, L., Dauser, C., Warnick, E., Scahill, L., Chakir, A. R., Shechner, T., & Hermes, H. (2013). Family accommodation in pediatric anxiety disorders. *Depression and Anxiety, 30*(1), 47–54. https://doi.org/10.1002/da.21998

Lewin, A. B., McGuire, J. F., Murphy, T. K., & Storch, E. A. (2014). Editorial perspective: The importance of considering parent's preferences when planning treatment for their children—the case of childhood obsessive-compulsive disorder. *Journal of Child Psychology and Psychiatry, 55*(12), 1314–1316. https://doi.org/10.1111/jcpp.12344

Lewin, A. B., Park, J. M., Jones, A. M., Crawford, E. A., De Nadai, A. S., Menzel, J., Arnold, E. B., Murphy, T. K., & Storch, E. A. (2014). Family-based exposure and response prevention therapy for preschool-aged children with obsessive-compulsive disorder: A pilot randomized controlled trial. *Behaviour Research and Therapy, 56*, 30–38. https://doi.org/10.1016/j.brat.2014.02.001

McGuire, J. F., Piacentini, J., Lewin, A. B., Brennan, E. A., Murphy, T. K., & Storch, E. A. (2015). A meta-analysis of cognitive behavior therapy and medication for child obsessive-compulsive disorder: Moderators of treatment efficacy, response, and remission. *Depression and Anxiety, 32*(8), 580–593. https://doi.org/10.1002/da.22389

McKay, M. M., & Bannon, W. M. (2004). Engaging families in child mental health services. *Child and Adolescent Psychiatric Clinics of North America, 13*(4), 905–921. https://doi.org/10.1016/j.chc.2004.04.001

Parsons, T. D., Riva, G., Parsons, S., Mantovani, F., Newbutt, N., Lin, L., Venturini, E., & Hall, T. (2017). Virtual reality in pediatric psychology. *Pediatrics, 140*, 86–91. https://doi.org/10.1542/peds.2016-1758I

Peris, T. S., Storch, E. A., & McGuire, J. F. (Eds.). (2020). *Exposure therapy for children with anxiety and OCD: Clinician's guide to integrated treatment*. Academic Press.

Peterman, J. S., Carper, M. M., & Kendall, P. C. (2019). Testing the habituation-based model of exposures for child and adolescent anxiety. *Journal of Clinical Child & Adolescent Psychology, 48*(Supp 1), S34–S44. https://doi.org/10.1080/15374416.2016.1163707

Peterman, J. S., Read, K. L., Wei, C., & Kendall, P. C. (2015). The art of exposure: Putting science into practice. *Cognitive and Behavioral Practice, 22*(3), 379–392. https://doi.org/10.1016/j.cbpra.2014.02.003

Rauch, S. A. M., & Foa, E. B. (2006). Emotional processing theory and exposure therapy for PTSD. *Journal of Contemporary Psychotherapy, 36*, 61–67. https://doi.org/10.1007/s10879-006-9008-y

Richard, D. C. S., & Gloster, A. T. (2007). Exposure therapy has a public relations problem: A dearth of litigation amid a wealth of concern. In D. C. S. Richard & D. Lauterbach (Eds.), *Handbook of exposure therapies* (pp. 409–429). Elsevier.

Rudy, B. M., Zavrou, S., Johnco, C., Storch, E. A., & Lewin, A. B. (2017). Parent-led exposure therapy: A pilot study of a brief behavioral treatment for anxiety in young children. *Journal of Child and Family Studies, 26*(9), 2475–2484. https://doi.org/10.1007/s10826-017-0772-y

Salloum A., Robst J., Scheeringa M. S., Cohen J. A., Wang W., Murphy T. K., Tolin D. F., & Storch, E. A. (2014). Step one within stepped care trauma-focused cognitive behavioral therapy for young children: A pilot study. *Child Psychiatry and Human Development, 45*, 65–77. https://doi.org/10.1007/s10578-013-0378-6

Salloum, A., Scheeringa, M. S., Cohen, J. A., & Storch, E. A. (2014). Development of stepped care trauma-focused cognitive-behavioral therapy for young children. *Cognitive and Behavioral Practice, 21*(1), 97–108. https://doi.org/10.1016/j.cbpra.2013.07.004

Saxe, G. N., Ellis, B. H., & Kaplow, J. B. (2007). *Collaborative treatment of traumatized children and teens: The trauma systems therapy approach*. Guilford Press.

Schneider, S. C., Knott, L., Cepeda, S. L., Hana, L. M., McIngvale, E., Goodman, W. K., & Storch, E. A. (2020). Serious negative consequences associated with exposure and response prevention for obsessive-compulsive disorder: A survey of therapist attitudes and experiences. *Depression and Anxiety, 37*(5), 418–428. https://doi.org/10.1002/da.23000

Shi, Q., & Brown, M. H. (2020). School counselors' impact on school-level academic outcomes: Caseload and use of time. *Professional School Counseling, 23*(1 part 3), 1–8. https://doi.org/10.1177/2156759X20904489

Silverman, W. K., Ortiz, C. D., Chockalingham, V., Burns, B. J., Kolko, D. J., Putnam, F. W., & Amaya-Jackson, L. (2008). Evidence-based psychosocial treatments for children and adolescents exposed to traumatic events. *Journal of Clinical Child & Adolescent Psychology, 37*(1), 156–183. https://doi.org/10.1080/15374416.2016.1220309

Storch, E. A., Arnold, E. B., Lewin, A. B., Nadeau, J. M., Jones, A. M., De Nadai, A. S., Mutch, P. J., Selles, R. S., Ung, D., & Murphy, T. K. (2013). The effect of cognitive-behavioral therapy versus treatment as usual for anxiety in children with autism spectrum disorders: A randomized, controlled trial. *Journal of the American Academy of Child & Adolescent Psychiatry, 52*(2), 132–142. https://doi.org/10.1016/j.jaac.2012.11.007

Storch, E. A., Geffken, G. R., Merlo, L. J., Jacob, M. L., Murphy, T. K., Goodman, W. K., Larson, M. J., Fernandez, M., & Grabill, K. (2007). Family accommodation in pediatric obsessive-compulsive disorder. *Journal of Clinical Child and Adolescent Psychology, 36*(2), 207–216. https://doi.org/10.1080/15374410701277929

Sukhodolsky, D. G., Bloch, M. H., Panza, K. E., & Reichow, B. (2013). Cognitive-behavioral therapy for anxiety in children with high-functioning autism: A meta-analysis. *Pediatrics, 132*(5), 1341–1350. https://doi.org/10.1542/peds.2013-1193

Tiwari, S., Kendall, P. C., Hoff, A. L., Harrison, J. P., & Fizur, P. (2013). Characteristics of exposure sessions as predictors of treatment response in anxious youth. *Journal of Clinical Child & Adolescent Psychology, 42*(1), 34–43. https://doi.org/10.1080/15374416.2012.738454

Tryon, W. W. (2008). Whatever happened to symptom substitution? *Clinical Psychology Review, 28*, 963–968. https://doi.org/10.1016/j.cpr.2008.02.003

Vande Voort, J. L. V., Svecova, J., Jacobson, A. B., & Whiteside, S. P. (2010). A retrospective examination of the similarity between clinical practice and manualized treatment for childhood anxiety disorders. *Cognitive and Behavioral Practice, 17*(3), 322–328. https://doi.org/10.1016/j.cbpra.2009.12.002

Wang, Z., Whiteside, S. P., Sim, L., Farah, W., Morrow, A. S., Alsawas, M., Barrionuevo, P., Tello, M., Asi, N., Beuschel, B., Daraz, L., Almasri, J., Zaiem, F., Larrea-Mantilla, F., Ponce, O. J., LeBlanc, A., Prokop, L. J., & Murad, M. H. (2017). Comparative effectiveness and safety of cognitive behavioral therapy and pharmacotherapy for childhood anxiety disorders: A systematic review and meta-analysis. *JAMA Pediatrics, 171*(11), 1049–1056. https://doi.org/10.1001/jamapediatrics.2017.3036

Weist, M. D., Eber, L., Horner, R., Splett, J., Putnam, R., Barrett, S., Perales, K., Fairchild, A. J., & Hoover, S. (2018). Improving multitiered systems of support for students with "internalizing" emotional/behavioral problems. *Journal of Positive Behavior Interventions, 20*(3), 172–184. https://doi.org/10.1177/1098300717753832

Wolpe, J. (1958). *Psychotherapy by reciprocal inhibition*. Stanford University Press.

Wood, J. J., Drahota, A., Sze, K., Har, K., Chiu, A., & Langer, D. A. (2009). Cognitive behavioral therapy for anxiety in children with autism spectrum disorders: A randomized, controlled trial. *Journal of Child Psychology and Psychiatry, 50*(3), 224–234. https://doi.org/10.1111/j.1469-7610.2008.01948.x

Wood, J. J., Kendall, P. C., Wood, K. S., Kerns, C. M., Seltzer, M., Small, B. J., Lewin, A. B., & Storch, E. A. (2019). Cognitive behavioral treatments for anxiety in children with autism spectrum disorder: A randomized clinical trial. *JAMA Psychiatry, 77*(5), 1–10. https://doi.org/10.1001/jamapsychiatry.2019.4160

Yasinski, C., Hayes, A., Alpert, E., McCauley, T., Ready, C. B, Webbs, C., & Deblinger, E. (2018). Treatment processes and demographic variables as predictors of dropout from trauma-focused cognitive behavioral therapy (TF-CBT) for youth. *Behavior Research & Therapy, 107*, 10–18. https://doi.org/10.1016/j.brat.2018.05.008

Yasinski, C., Hayes, A. M., Ready, C. B., Cummings, J. A., Berman, I. S., McCauley, T., Webb, C., & Deblinger, E. (2016). In-session caregiver behavior predicts symptom change in youth receiving trauma-focused cognitive behavioral therapy (TF-CBT). *Journal of Consulting and Clinical Psychology, 84*(12), 1066–1077. https://doi.org/10.1037/ccp0000147

Zaboski, B. A. (2020). Exposure therapy for anxiety disorders in schools: Getting started. *Contemporary School Psychology,* Article 144. https://doi.org/10.1007/s40688-020-00301-0

Zaboski, B. A., Joyce-Beaulieu, D., Kranzler, J. H., McNamara, J. P., Gayle, C., & MacInnes, J. (2019). Group exposure and response prevention for college students with social anxiety: A randomized clinical trial. *Journal of Clinical Psychology, 75*(9), 1489–1507. https://doi.org/10.1002/jclp.22792

Zaboski, B. A., & Storch, E. A. (2018). Comorbid autism spectrum disorder and anxiety disorders: A brief review. *Future Neurology, 13*(1), 31–37. https://doi.org/10.2217/fnl-2017-0030

8

Integrating Technology into School-Based Interventions

GREG M. MULLER, BRIAN A. ZABOSKI,
AND DIANA JOYCE-BEAULIEU ■

A RATIONALE FOR INCORPORATING TECHNOLOGY IN PRACTICE

From the Victorian daybed of Sigmund Freud to the audiovisual casting software in contemporary telehealth practices, therapy tools have had a long history of development. Since the innovation of cellular devices and mobile applications (apps), therapists have attempted to integrate these technologies into their clinical practice (e.g., Evans et al., 2013). However, the use of mobile applications also has value in school-based interventions, for example through behavioral tracking, teaching mindfulness/relaxation strategies, and broadening the availability of self-help resources. This chapter reviews the development and efficacy of technology and mobile apps for school-based practice, discusses their applicability in school-based interventions, and highlights usage barriers. For convenience, "mobile apps" will refer generally to apps that run on the Apple operating system (iOS) and Android devices.

Most school-based providers are already using technology as part of their interventions and daily activities, like drafting comprehensive assessments through word processors, scoring omnibus and single-construct measures with web-based software, scheduling appointments through electronic calendars, and communicating with coworkers through email. Additional technology available to school-based providers includes behavioral intervention technologies (BITs). Broadly defined, BITs are treatment-augmenting technologies within behavioral/psychological interventions that enhance a student's functioning (Burns & Mohr, 2013; Mohr et al., 2013). Evidence-based examples from the literature include computerized cognitive behavioral therapy (CBT) for anxiety (Ben-Moussa et al.,

2017; Ebert et al., 2015; Jones et al., 2016; Pennant et al., 2015; Urech et al., 2015; Zidani, et al., 2017), depression (Ebert et al., 2015; Pennant et al., 2015), and stress management (Winslow et al., 2016). There are more specific applications, too, like physiological data collection through the Biopac MP-150 system and mHealth mobile app (Winslow et al., 2016). A more sophisticated BIT, virtual reality, is used for treatment plans that include exposure and response prevention to simulate environments that cannot be easily accessed within an educational or traditional outpatient setting (e.g., flying on an airplane to address a fear of heights; Inozu et al., 2020).

Mobile phones are an increasingly relevant BIT. The most pertinent distinction between mobile operating systems (mOS) is among Android (Android, Inc.) and iOS (Apple, Inc.). Operating systems are preinstalled instructions that allow a device to coordinate software (programs installed on a device) with hardware (e.g., the parts of a phone), allowing the user to execute important functions (e.g., start the device; University of Wolongong, 2019). A mobile device's operating system is designed to function similarly to a desktop computer, with architecture that supports an on-the-go interface (e.g., a touchscreen) and mobile storefronts (App Store iOS; Google Play) that allow users to download apps (Apple Inc., 2020; Google LLC, 2020). Apps are programs that allow users to execute specific actions (e.g., checking social media) on a device. Apps vary widely by genre: entertainment, communication, organization, physical health, lifestyles, shopping, education, etc.

Following iPhone 1's release in 2007, smartphone technology has become more widely accessible to the public, allowing practitioners to more readily integrate mobile apps within behavioral interventions (Grossman, 2007). Anderson and Jiang (2018) suggests that 95% of U.S. teenagers own a smartphone. Researchers at the Pew Research Center note that these trends are "nearly universal among teens of different genders, races and ethnicities and socioeconomic backgrounds" (Anderson & Jiang, 2018, "Vast majority of teens" section). An online survey of 500 women suggests that ownership occurs early, with an average age for receiving a first phone at 10.3 years (Influence Central, 2016). These findings are corroborated by a nonprofit firm, Common Sense, whose representative, cross-sectional survey of 8- to 18-year-olds found that smartphone ownership happens early and grows fast: 53% at age 11, 69% at age 12, and 72% by age 13 (Rideout & Robb, 2019). Because of early and ubiquitous smartphone ownership, we recommend that practitioners leverage technological advances to create sustainable school-based interventions.

THE THERAPEUTIC BENEFITS OF APPS

Having substantiated the widespread use of technology in the schools, a legitimate question remains: "What benefit does this technology offer beyond traditional psychotherapy?"

First, technology can assist providers to meet rising demands for mental health services. Consider that approximately one in six children in the United States experiences a mental health condition, with nearly half of children with a treatable mental health disorder not receiving treatment (Whitney & Peterson, 2019). Moreover, suicide is the second leading cause of death for school-aged youth (Nguyen & Davis, 2017), and depression is the leading cause of disability within global adolescent populations, impacting functioning and quality of life into adulthood (World Health Organization, 2019). Thus, widely available technology allows practitioners to reach more students in need before they develop untreated or refractory symptoms.

Second, technology can address the nationwide shortage of mental health providers. Although the National Association of School Psychologists (2019) advocates for a ratio of 1 school psychologist per 500 to 700 students, they estimate a current ratio of 1:1,381. Another report suggests that there are only 30 general psychologists per 100,000 individuals, and in nonmetropolitan areas 47% of U.S. counties lack any psychologist at all (Andrilla et al., 2018). Consequently, together the high need for and dearth of mental health professionals has innervated discussion on using technology as an easily disseminated access-to-care solution.

Third, mobile app-based interventions are a no- to low-cost solution that allow students to access resources that reinforce their counseling sessions. For instance, a school psychologist who teaches and models mindfulness-based stress reduction strategies may recommend a mobile app that provides a student with daily reminders to practice box breathing and that tracks assignment completion. Some apps also have supplemental or more detailed instructions that review what students have learned in a counseling session (e.g., a step-by-step procedure for grounding techniques). By incorporating technology into an intervention, the provider coordinates care and monitors the student's progress as they practice these strategies at home. Of note, we do not recommend that apps supplant the role of the therapist; rather, we recommend their use as therapeutic aids that allow clients to review material and practice techniques outside of session (Raento et al., 2009).

Fourth, by their nature mobile applications are portable, and students are reluctant to lose their phones, increasing opportunities to access care. Consequently, counselors can worry less about printed therapy materials getting lost in a backpack or eaten by the proverbial dog. Some concerns about a caregiver's ability to attend school-based appointments are also addressed, as therapy materials can be reviewed with their child anywhere, anytime. Mobile apps also offer an alternative way to monitor progress rather than relying on a student's recollection of their behavior or on paper copies that can be misplaced. Behavior tracking apps such as Daylio (Habitics, 2020; Relaxio S.R.O., 2020) or Habit-bull (AppForge Inc., 2020; App Holdings, 2020) can provide timed reminders for students to participate in therapy assignments. This feature may increase homework completion and facilitate data acquisition in treatment-relevant contexts (e.g., subjective stress ratings at school/home, completion of math coursework during school hours). Mobile phone apps also facilitate longitudinal data collection (Mays et al., 2010) from large samples of students/clients at a reduced cost (Raento et al., 2009). Taken together, mobile apps can help school-based personnel triage students who (a) require more scaffolding to reach mastery criteria with therapy skills, (b) progress at an adequate rate toward their intervention goals, or (c) may not be adequately engaged.

Lastly, mobile apps relieve providers from having to aggregate progress-monitoring results and provide quick and meaningful data visualizations. Providers can interpret data during therapy sessions to determine whether to modify treatment or to use the data in team meetings to discuss students' progress. Additionally, these data can be leveraged to praise hard work and build rapport. Moreover, for clients who struggle with maladaptive cognitions (e.g., discounting the positive, see Chapter 6), these results can be an opportunity to examine the evidence and to challenge such thinking errors.

MOBILE APP CONSIDERATIONS

The best mobile app to use in a behavioral intervention program will depend on the student's presenting concerns. For individuals experiencing significant deficits in mathematics fluency, apps that build fluency through game-based programming (e.g., "race the clock" to earn in-app currency) may be most appropriate. Alternatively, students seeking to build self-efficacy can download programs that provide daily affirmations. School-based therapists can also select specific apps to target therapy goals, such as mobile journals. While these applications are not a substitute for individualized therapy, they may enhance established treatment plans.

Additional considerations for selecting a mobile app include cost and a student's developmental level. Mobile apps range from no- to low-cost pricing to recurring monthly/annual subscriptions. A top-of-the-line app that does not match one's financial circumstances may be unhelpful. Thus, when selecting an app, balance the benefits offered by free programs with the features offered by more expensive apps. Many mobile apps require the user to be independent, so students with significant difficulties (e.g., intellectual disabilities) might find certain apps frustrating. These individuals may require educators to scaffold the use of the app, might need a modified app interface, or simply use an alternative to mobile intervention technologies. Considering these goodness-of-fit factors, evaluate mobile apps based on user reviews, popularity, and demonstrated efficacy. A benefit of more popular apps is that they likely (a) have greater technical support by the manufacturer, (b) continue to expand/refine their features, and (c) are familiar to a community of professionals. This final point implies that one should consider intervention apps familiar to coworkers to support the intervention team's cohesion.

Many mobile apps also incorporate social media features within their interfaces. This may provide the opportunity to highlight student progress in classroom/group therapy settings; however, limitations relate to student privacy or peer hostility.

Mobile apps with social media features can be monitored and prescreened by a professional therapist for content, and inappropriate comments can be removed. Some are monitored by an algorithm for toxic word content. Conversely, unmonitored apps may be vulnerable to malicious commenting. Consequently, before selecting an app, practitioners should understand how developers monitor social media interactions.

Another consideration is the extent to which the mobile app maintains student attention and increases engagement. Researchers have reported that gaming in childhood continues through adolescence, with a high prevalence among teens (72%), particularly males (84%) compared to females (59%; Fromme, 2003; Lenhart, 2015; Oblinger, 2004). Additionally, research indicates that "gamifying" or "gamification" of traditional instruction increases student engagement during activity breaks (Beemer et al., 2019). One popular application is Kahoot!, a game-based educational program used by half of U.S. students (Luden, 2018). Other researchers have reported effective use of gamified technologies within clinical samples to treat anxiety (Ben-Moussa et al., 2017). Overall, research shows that merging games with school-based interventions increases student interest, may be particularly well suited for male clients, and shows promise in some clinical populations.

Although an exhaustive review of the mobile marketplace is beyond this chapter's scope, the following sections provide an entry point for practitioners wishing to use mobile apps in their practice.[1] To provide an organizational framework, we divided mobile apps into three categories: behavioral tracking, mindfulness/relaxation, and therapy/self-help. Behavioral tracking apps (BTAs) allow the individual to monitor progress toward a targeted goal. Mindfulness/relaxation-based apps support these therapeutic techniques through a variety of means, such as ambient music or guided imagery. Therapy/self-help is a broad category that captures any mobile app that offers general psychoeducation or scaffolds therapeutic skills.

Behavioral Tracking

Behavioral tracking apps (BTAs) can be general or specific. When selecting a BTA, consider whether a general or a specific app would better facilitate the intervention's goals. A general app allows for more customized tracking based on frequency and duration, granting users maximum freedom to specify complex goals across different domains. For instance, a practitioner could specify two goals: Engage in daily exercise and use grounding strategies at least three times per day. Specific BTAs tend to be preferrable for behaviors in a similar domain since users can rapidly generate goals from premade templates (e.g., For Habit-bull: "Add" > "Water" > " ___ cup(s)" per day > Done). Specific BTA categories include menstrual cycles (FLO HEALTH, INC., 2020a, 2020b); fitness (MyFitnessPal, Inc., 2020; MapMyFitness, 2020; Smillage, Inc., 2020; Under Armour Inc., 2020a, 2020b), medication management (Medisafe Inc., 2020a,

2020b), and diabetes management (One Drop, 2020; One Drop and Informed Data Systems Inc., 2020).

Several studies have established the efficacy of BTAs. One pilot study examining the health tracking behaviors of 10- to 12-year-olds reported an enhanced ability to examine their social habits, living environments, and other recurring behaviors (Sormunen & Miettinen, 2017). BTAs are also efficacious for tracking behaviors in individuals on the autism spectrum (Bangerter et al., 2019) and for weight loss in overweight/obese adults (Hales et al., 2016). They have also been recommended for monitoring socially or geographically isolated populations (e.g., men recently released from prison), highlighting their potential to increase participation rates (Sugie, 2018).

Two general BTAs, Habit-bull and Productive (IAC Search & Media Technologies Limited, 2020), are available on the iOS and Android operating systems. These applications are freeware (openly available software) at no cost. Both applications allow the therapist to set general goals (e.g., "other" and "regular habit") or specify goals from a series of options (e.g., Arts, Health & Fitness, Money, Work & Study, Learn & Explore). One can then customize the type of tracking needed. For instance, Habit-bull includes tracking the goal discretely (yes/no) or quantitatively (e.g., drank 2 cans of soda today). To aid in progress monitoring, users may also select a target date or number of days-to-success to complete a goal. Habit-bull has options for adjusting the interval (e.g., a goal recurring on Wednesdays; drawing at least twice per day), and Productive offers similar features with a more intuitive interface. In both apps, aesthetics can also be modified (e.g., the goal's avatar, color scheme). Some limitations include monthly subscription fees to access optimal features; for example, Productive has additional goal reminders based on one's location. Likewise, the free version of Habit-bull restricts the number of goals to 5, while Habit-bull Premium allows up to 100. While these premium features are preferable, forgoing them does not necessarily impede intervention quality.

BTAs also provide a means for practitioners to collaborate with outside professionals. For instance, a majority of students prescribed medications do not take them routinely (Rapoff, 2010), and 6.1 million U.S. youths have been diagnosed with attention-deficit/hyperactivity disorder (Centers for Disease Control and Prevention, 2019). Yet a study of 2,206 pediatric youth found that only 46% of them adhered to their stimulants (Biederman et al., 2019). As such, school-based mental health workers can collaborate with other professionals through BTAs to increase medication adherence. One helpful app, Medisafe, prompts users to enter the medication's name, dosage/units, and appearance (e.g., capsule vs. injectable; medication color) and are prompted to set reminder frequency (Medisafe Inc., 2020b). There is also the option to add details related to the medication's purpose, prescription number, volume of medication remaining, and refill reminders. Users then input their behavioral tracking goals (i.e., medication taken "Now"; "On Time"; "Set Time"). Through close tracking and monitoring, school psychologists can help limit adverse side effects from inconsistent medication use. Additionally, these apps can improve communication between school and medical staff.

See Quick Resource 8.1 in the Appendix for a list of behavioral tracking and intervention apps.

Mindfulness and Relaxation

Mindfulness includes practices that help practitioners develop self-compassion and present-minded awareness of their thoughts, sensations, and environment (see Chapter 3). Mindfulness practices are varied but typically include mindful breathing, body scanning, and behaviors that facilitate meditation (e.g., walking, loving-kindness). Behavioral health providers also employ various mindfulness protocols, including mindfulness-based stress reduction and mindfulness-based cognitive therapy.

Contemporary apps that support mindfulness-based interventions include Headspace (Headspace Inc., 2020a, 2020b), Calm (Calm.com, Inc., 2020a, 2020b), and Waking Up: A Meditation Course (Waking Up LLC, 2020a, 2020b). After installation, Headspace directs users to select a priority: managing anxiety/stress, sleep, physical activity, or doing something new. The app also offers introductory audio presentations on the foundations of mindfulness, as well as content-specific resources like narrated guided imagery scripts, visualizations, and ambient noises/tones for sleep. Headspace also includes mindful exercise routines with various cardio/strength trainings and rest-day meditations. To manage stress, users can even select from narrated mindfulness courses and then watch animated videos to practice new skills.

An alternative to Headspace, Calm has similar features with introductory/advanced mindfulness trainings and sleep hygiene practices. Calm uniquely includes a "breathe bubble," an animated circle that guides users through the processes of mindful breathing, and Sleep Stories: celebrity audio recordings from Bob Ross, Eva Green, and Nick Offerman (to name a few). Calm also features daily behavior tracking for mood (e.g., ecstatic, relaxed, anxious, angry).

Developed by neuroscientist Sam Harris, Waking Up: A Meditation Course advertises two functions: to practice meditation and to learn the underlying theory (Waking Up LLC, 2020a). To that end, Dr. Harris provides a series of brief audios that introduce mindfulness theory and different forms of practice. Unique features of Waking Up are "groups" (with a premium account) to engage in synchronized meditation with other users. Additionally, the app provides a timer to structure meditations (e.g., discrete time, or in intervals). Of note, Dr. Harris has openly invited anyone who cannot afford the app to email him for discounted or free access.

Two other mobile applications for relaxation, Spotify (Spotify Ltd., 2020a, 2020b) and A Soft Murmur (Polarised Light Ltd., 2020; Sleepy Rabbit LLC, 2020), are worth discussing. Spotify is a multi-genre audio streaming service founded in 2006. The platform hosts a tremendous breadth of content, including music, podcasts, and lectures, from which users can also browse guided imagery scripts and ambient noises. Podcasters on mindfulness can also be found for both religious (e.g., Be Here Now Network, 2020) and secular (e.g., Harris, 2020) interests. With its user-friendly interface, A Soft Murmur app sets and blends a variety of ambient noises (e.g., rain, fire, crickets, wind) to reduce distress and aid focus.

Incorporating mobile apps into mindfulness training is easy. In addition to psychoeducation and traditional CBT strategies, providers can assist the student in downloading an app that matches their intervention goals. Students with racing thoughts can utilize A Soft Murmur to provide distraction or can listen to a Headspace lecture (e.g., Managing Anxiety). Apps like Calm can offer a quasi-manualized treatment approach for homework. For example, students can complete specific modules that can then be discussed during the next session (e.g., "Radical Self-Compassion" from Calm). Consider this general plan:

Session 1: Mindfulness psychoeducation; review of body scans.
Session 1—Homework: View/practice Headspace's Body Scan content.
Session 2: Review content from Headspace and then model/practice body scans in session.

Despite their user-friendly formats, a significant barrier with Headspace and Calm is the need for a recurring monthly subscription for premium content. While mindfulness/relaxation-based applications augment behavioral intervention efforts, students may find these costs unappealing. As such, providers are encouraged to discuss these limitations with students and caregivers. Although Spotify and A Soft Murmur permit greater accessibility, they may lack targeted intervention content (e.g., a meditation timer). Providers should collaborate with the student in selecting the app that targets their needs most efficiently while considering these drawbacks. See Quick Resource 8.2 in the Appendix for a list of mindfulness and relaxation-based apps.

Therapy/Self-Help

Therapy/self-help apps can be paired with BTAs and mindfulness-based apps in a polytherapy approach. To streamline student access to educational and therapy materials, Kindle (Amazon.com, Inc., 2020; Amazon Mobile LLC, 2020) and Quizlet (Quizlet, Inc., 2020a, 2020b) are two options. Developed by the marketing giant Amazon, Kindle is an e-reading program that allows users to purchase and read various digital media (e.g., books, magazines). Students can use it during sessions, throughout the school day, or at home to access psychoeducation materials or a therapy workbook (e.g., Tompkins & Martinez, 2010). Quizlet is a study-based application known for its learning tools (flashcards in particular). This application could help students with academic difficulties, improve their learning, and reduce distress.

Integrating mobile therapy apps into teacher consultation may also be advantageous. For example, if a teacher and practitioner hope to increase a socially anxious child's participation in class, they might use an app to track how often a student raises their hand in class. Several options include ClassDojo (ClassDojo, Inc., 2020a, 2020b), Bloomz (Bloomz Inc., 2020a, 2020b), and Time Timer (Time Timer, LLC, 2020a, 2020b). To improve communication between students, educators, and family members, ClassDojo is a popular resource. It allows educators to provide instant feedback to students and parents that can later be shared with the school psychologist. An alternative program, Bloomz, offers similar features. Time Timer presents a visual reminder of the remaining length of an activity, lesson, or therapy session and may be suitable for students who struggle with transitions. Teachers can use the app and later discuss the results with the student's counselor.

Started in 2005, YouTube (Google Inc., 2020) is the flagship video-streaming service on the internet. YouTube offers an extensive variety of psychoeducational content that can support students outside of session. Examples of relevant YouTube channels range from content specific (e.g., Headspace) to those that broadly discuss psychotherapy (e.g., CrashCourse, 2014; Grande, 2019). Potential limitations of YouTube include that students may consume entertainment content at the cost of productivity, and that subjective well-being may be negatively impacted by responses within a video's comment section. As discussed before, we encourage practitioners to consider the potential benefits and drawbacks of media that have social features (e.g., YouTube's comments section).

Students with specific concerns may benefit from targeted mobile applications. Suicidal ideation can be addressed through the Suicide Safety Plan (MoodTools, 2020a, 2020b) and My3 (CalMHSA, 2020; MHA-NYC, 2020) apps. The Suicide Safety Plan offers a plain interface that provides a straightforward way to establish care. Users list warning signs, coping strategies, reasons to live, designated safety contacts (e.g., parent), distracting places, and other safety behaviors. My3 offers similar features, with a greater emphasis on the three individuals the user designates on their safety plan. My3 emails the user's safety plan (i.e., to their therapist) and pins resources on the app dashboard (e.g., the Trevor Project website for LGBTQ+ youth; Trevor Project, 2020).

We have two suggestions for older students with substance-related or addiction problems: I Am Sober (I Am Sober LLC, 2020a, 2020b) and SoberTool (Blitzen, LLC, 2020). On the former, the student selects what they wish to abstain from. This includes traditional (e.g., alcohol, tobacco, cocaine, gambling) and nontraditional (e.g., sugar, videogames, sex) habits. They can specify their date of sobriety, the daily financial cost of engaging in the habit, and reasons for wanting to abstain. From the main menu, I Am Sober has a clock that tracks how long the user was successful. The app also displays a calculation of how much money and time the student is saving. Additionally, I Am Sober offers a pledge feature so users can abstain for prespecified intervals (e.g., 24 hours; 7 days). I Am Sober also has some gamification like milestones that are unlocked after certain timepoints (e.g., day 1; double digits). A social media menu allows the student to post with other users, explore motivational packs that provide daily quotes (e.g., from Aristotle), and find licensed therapists. SoberTool offers comparable features to I Am Sober with a unique navigational menu that provides abstinence resource flowcharts that direct users to positive activities (e.g., Need motivation? > Do you feel hopeless? > Try "Surviving Riptides" and a related "To Do" activity).

Some apps are a great developmental fit for younger school-aged children or those with low-incidence disabilities (e.g., autism spectrum disorders), communication difficulties, or adaptive/social skills needs. Two options are the First-Then Visual Schedule (Good Karma Applications, Inc., 2020) and iReward (Grembe Apps Inc., 2020) apps. First-Then helps build structure with visual schedules, which can help increase student autonomy and assist with daily transitions (Pierce et al., 2013). iReward has star and/or token boards to reinforce positive behaviors. iReward can also be used for more general problems, such as concentration difficulties, anxiety, and depression. While these apps can be used on mobile phones, the visual schedules may be clearer on a tablet.

Several options can help students manage their time, and Focus Keeper (HSM Studio, 2020; PIXO Inc., 2020), Flora (AppFinca Inc., 2020), and Study Bunny (Silang, 2020; SuperByte, 2020) are more than just clockfaces. Focus Keeper tracks 25-minute intervals of continuous work, with subsequent 5-minute breaks. These values represent advised intervals but can be adjusted. With Flora, students plant a virtual tree that grows within the menu the longer the user remains active. If the user returns to the phone's home screen, the tree "dies." The app also allows users to link their credit card to the account and risk real-world money (i.e., a response cost) if they "kill" a tree (according to the app's website, the money is used to plant trees in the real world). This feature may benefit older adolescents or college-age students looking for extrinsic motivation to remain engaged. Lastly, an example of a timer with gamified features is Study Bunny. Users are given a cartoon rabbit that they can name and give unique items by redeeming coins (e.g., hat, glasses). Coins are earned for every 10 minutes the user studies while using the app. The program also provides study aids, including a to-do list and flashcards. See Quick Resource 8.3 in the Appendix for therapy and self-help apps.

LIMITATIONS OF MOBILE APPS

While there are definite advantages for utilizing mobile apps, it is necessary to consider their limitations, including the research base supporting particular types of apps. Primarily, utilizing mobile apps depends on a student's access to cellular devices. First, while the research discussed in this chapter demonstrates that students are receiving phones at young ages, this is not universal. Students from low socioeconomic backgrounds may have more limited access. For schools that issue Chromebooks or similar devices to all students, administrators might consider purchasing broad usage contracts that would permit access to specific apps for all of their students. Additionally, parents may not wish some children to have a cellphone out of monetary or safety concerns, and premium features can complicate monetary considerations. Second, mobile devices must be powered to work, which may limit access to content during critical circumstances (e.g., accessing My3's safety plan when in crisis and on low battery). As such, school-based providers are encouraged to provide multimodal resources (i.e., paper and electronic copies).

Third, school policy may restrict students' access to cellphones during school hours. School-based providers must be aware of these logistic restrictions and advocate on their students' behalf; for example, they might request formal accommodations for access during the school day. Lastly, success in using mobile apps depends on the provider's and student's fluency with technology. Before integrating mobile apps within treatment, providers must consider their expertise at using these technologies; furthermore, they should not assume knowledge on the student's part. Installing and navigating app features should be included in session activities before assigning apps as homework. Several national agencies provide online reviews and guidance on apps with supportive research that meet best practice standards (e.g., Northwestern University's Center for Behavioral Intervention Technologies, National Center for Telehealth and Technology, iMedicalApps, Center for Technology in Behavioral Science, and the Anxiety and Depression Association of America Mobile App Clearinghouse).

TECHNOLOGY CASE STUDY

This case study illustrates how to incorporate mobile app technologies into the therapeutic process.

Claire is a 13-year-old female referred to the school psychologist for falling asleep in class. Her teachers report that Claire has difficulty paying attention during lessons and that her grades have been steadily falling over the past semester. She is rarely seen socializing with her classmates and eats lunch alone in the cafeteria.

There are a variety of ways to incorporate mobile apps within school-based interventions. The most relevant consideration is matching the presenting concern to the indicated mobile intervention class (e.g., BTA, mindfulness/relaxation-based, or therapy/self-help). BTAs represent an effective starting point for most concerns. School-based providers are encouraged to first assess the student's behaviors of concern:

> THERAPIST What should we focus on during our sessions?
> CLAIRE I just feel miserable. Any little thing sets me off, and I can't pay attention during class.
> T How much sleep do you get most nights?
> C Um . . . I'm not sure. It depends on how much work I get and if people are texting me.
> T That makes sense; many students struggle with sleep. Do you like apps? We can start with Daylio. It'll give us a bunch of information that'll help.

c OK. I could try that.

From these data, the provider can select intervention targets and establish baselines. A subsequent session might progress as follows:

t How's this week been going so far?
c Good. I used Daylio.
t And?
c Well, even though I'm in bed by 10, I'm not done texting til 1.
t So, being tired during the school day makes sense. How can we change this?
c Hmm, that's what I'm stuck on.
t That's OK; I think I can help. Maybe we should talk about sleep hygiene. Ever hear of it?

Having established the use of a BTA, the provider can assign sleep hygiene homework for the student to track (e.g., put the phone away by 10:30 p.m., keep it in another room before bed, entrust the phone to a parent/guardian before bed). Using BTAs consistently allows stakeholders and students to monitor the intervention's success. This approach can also facilitate meaningful discussions with the student related to success ("What about this worked for you?") or stuck points ("What made your homework challenging?").

Mindfulness and relaxation-based mobile apps help students engage in daily practice. When introducing mindfulness content, it may be important to address common hesitations or concerns:

t So, we talked about it before, but what are your thoughts on mindfulness?
c Honestly? It seems dumb. Breathing won't make my problems go away. I just get more anxious as I sit there.

Validate and normalize the student's concerns. Also consider showing its effectiveness by linking it to hobbies (e.g., for sports, LeBron James's use of mindfulness). By building rapport and increasing the relevance of the intervention to the student, one can also introduce a mobile app into treatment:

c I've been SO anxious this week! We have state testing and I just can't deal.
t What makes this testing harder than usual?
c The pressure! And, well, I have trouble remembering the mindfulness stuff.
t What would make remembering easier?
c I don't know; I just have trouble remembering to do the meditating.
t Hmmm. There's an app called Waking Up that lets you set reminders and has a timer that lets you know when you are finished.
c Oh cool! That'd make this a lot easier—I always have my phone with me anyway.

When teaching mindfulness-based practices, we recommend that providers thoroughly model the skills in session and then encourage students to practice them independently. Therapy/self-help apps have the broadest applications of the three intervention app categories. It is worth considering combining multiple apps to create a polytherapy approach. For example:

T Have you noticed any changes in your mood this week?
C Yeah . . . I just feel like everything's a total waste. I just want to fall asleep and have my problems go away (tearful affect).
T Wow, that's a lot to deal with. You've said similar things before when you've had thoughts about hurting yourself. Is that going on right now?
C (nods head) I don't want to, and I told my parents . . . I just feel so alone.
T Remember our safety plan that we worked on? Let's take another look, and this time we'll put it in an app so that you always have it.
C We can do that?
T Absolutely! We can use this My3 app. You'll always have help nearby.
C OK.
T Great. In your last safety plan, you mentioned that reading makes you feel better. Let's download Kindle too and get some of your favorite books set up.

CHAPTER DISCUSSION QUESTIONS

1. How would mobile behavioral intervention apps most impact your practice? What limitations exist for their use at your practicum/internship site?
2. What is your current comfort level with mobile apps? How might you go about remediating any related skill gaps?
3. A 13-year-old male presents with persistent concerns related to disruptive behaviors (e.g., aggression toward staff) and substance use. Which of the apps discussed in this chapter are indicated in supporting intervention efforts? How would you use them?
4. One of your client's teachers is unsupportive of using behavioral health apps during the school day. How might you advocate on your student's behalf to ensure access to care?
5. Write a sample treatment plan that blends traditional intervention practices with mobile apps to create multimodal care.
6. Mobile therapy apps require high accountability. How can school-based providers ensure that students utilize these resources outside of therapy?
7. What client characteristics (e.g., race, culture, socioeconomic status) might influence the utility of mobile apps in counseling?

NOTE

1. Note: For consistency throughout the text, we generally provide in-text citations for the iOS version of apps. We cite both iOS and Android versions in the References section.

REFERENCES

Amazon.com, Inc. (2020). *Kindle* (iOS Version 6.28) [Mobile Application Software]. App store. https://apps.apple.com/us/app/amazon-kindle/id302584613

Amazon Mobile LLC. (2020). *Kindle* (Varies with device) [Mobile Application Software]. Google Play. https://play.google.com/store/apps/details?id=com.amazon.kindle&hl=en_US

Anderson, M., & Jiang, J. (2018, May 31). Teens, social media & technology 2018. Pew Research Center. https://www.pewresearch.org/internet/2018/05/31/teens-social-media-technology-2018/

Andrilla, C. H., Patterson, D. G., Garberson, L. A., Coulthard, C., & Larson, E. H. (2018). Geographic variation in the supply of selected behavioral health providers. *American Journal of Preventative Medicine, 54*(6S3), S199–S207. https://doi.org/10.1016/j.amepre.2018.01.004

Apalon Apps. (2020). *Productive* (1.11.0) [Mobile Application Software]. Google Play. https://play.google.com/store/apps/details?id=com.apalon.to.do.list&hl=en_US

AppFinca Inc. (2020). *Flora* (iOs Version 2.5.19) [Mobile Application Software]. App store. https://apps.apple.com/us/app/flora-focus-habit-tracker/id1225155794

AppForge. (2020). *Habit-bull: Daily goal tracker* (iOS Version 1.3.5) [Mobile Application Software]. App store. https://apps.apple.com/us/app/habit-bull-daily-goal-tracker/id1041482672

App Holdings. (2020). *Habit-bull: Daily goal tracker* (1.5.11) [Mobile Application Software]. Google Play. https://play.google.com/store/apps/details?id=com.oristats.habitbull&hl=en_US

Apple Inc. (2020, April 20). *App Store Home Menu*. App Store (iOS). https://www.apple.com/ios/app-store/

Bangerter, A., Manyakov, N. V., Lewin, D., Boice, M., Skalkin, A., Jagannatha, S., Chatterjee, M., Dawson, G., Goodwin, M. S., Hendren, R., Leventhal, B., Shic, F., Ness, S., & Pandina, G. (2019). Caregiver daily reporting of symptoms in autism spectrum disorder: Observational study using web and mobile apps. *Journal of Medical Internet Research—Mental Health, 6*(3), Article e11365. https://doi.org/10.2196/11365

Beemer, L. R., Ajibewa, T. A., DellaVecchia, G., & Hasson, R. (2019). A pilot intervention using gamification to enhance student participation in classroom activity breaks. *International Journal of Research and Public Health, 16*(21), 1–11. https://doi.org/10.3390/ijerph16214082

Be Here Now Network. (2020). Ram Dass Here and Now Podcast [Audio podcast]. https://beherenownetwork.com/category/ram-dass/

Ben-Moussa, M., Rubo, M., Debracque, C., & Lange, W.-G. (2017). DJinni: A novel technology supported exposure therapy paradigm for SAD combining virtual reality and augmented reality. *Frontiers in Psychiatry, 8*(26), 1–12. https://doi.org/10.3389/fpsyt.2017.00026

Biederman, J., Fried, R., DiSalvo, M., Storch, B., Pulli, A., Woodworth, K. Y., Biederman, I., Faraone, S. V., & Perlis, R. H. (2019). Evidence of low adherence to stimulant medication among children and youths with ADHD: An electronic health records study. *Psychiatric Services, 70*(10), 874–880. https://doi.org/10.1176/appi.ps.20180051

Blitzen, LLC. (2020). *SoberTool* (iOS Version 4.2.2) [Mobile Application Software]. App store. https://apps.apple.com/us/app/sobertool-addiction-recovery/id863872931

Bloomz (2020a). *Bloomz* (3.22) [Mobile Application Software]. Google Play. https://play.google.com/store/apps/details?id=net.bloomz&hl=en_US

Bloomz Inc. (2020b). *Bloomz* (iOS Version 3.24) [Mobile Application Software]. App store. https://apps.apple.com/us/app/bloomz-for-teachers-schools/id690437499

Burns, M. N., & Mohr, D. C. (2013). eHealth and behavioral intervention technologies. In M. D. Gellman & J. R. Turner (Eds.), *Encyclopedia of behavioral medicine* (pp. 659–664). Springer. https://doi.org/10.1007/978-1-4419-1005-9_182

Calm.com, Inc. (2020a). *Calm* (iOS Version 4.22) [Mobile Application Software]. App Store. https://apps.apple.com/us/app/calm/id571800810

Calm.com, Inc. (2020b). *Calm* (Varies with device) [Mobile Application Software]. Google Play. https://play.google.com/store/apps/details?id=com.calm.android&hl=en_US

CalMHSA. (2020). *My3—Support Network* (iOS Version 5.2.0) [Mobile Application Software]. App store. https://apps.apple.com/us/app/my3-support-network/id709651264

Centers for Disease Control and Prevention. (2019, October 15). *Facts about ADHD*. https://www.cdc.gov/ncbddd/adhd/data.html

ClassDojo, Inc. (2020a). *ClassDojo* (iOS Version 6.22.0) [Mobile Application Software]. App store. https://apps.apple.com/us/app/classdojo/id552602056

ClassDojo, Inc. (2020b). *ClassDojo* (4.82.3) [Mobile Application Software]. Google Play. https://play.google.com/store/apps/details?id=com.classdojo.android&hl=en_US

CrashCourse. (2014). Getting Help—Psychotherapy: Crash Course Psychology #35 [Video file]. YouTube. https://www.youtube.com/watch?v=6nEL44QkL9w&list=PL8dPuuaLjXtOPRKzVLY0jJY-uHOH9KVU6&t=0s

Ebert, D. D., Zarski, A.-C., Christensen, H., Stikkelbroek, Cuijpers, P., Berking, M., & Riper, H. (2015). Internet and computer-based cognitive behavioral therapy for anxiety and depression in youth: A meta-analysis of randomized controlled outcome trials. *PLoS ONE, 10*(3), 1–15. https://doi.org/10.1371/journal.pone.0119895

Evans, W. P., Davison, L., & Sicafuse, L. (2013). Someone to listen: Increasing youth help-seeking behavior through a text-based crisis line for youth. *Journal of Community Psychology, 41*(4), 471–487. https://doi.org/10.1002/jcop.21551

FLO HEALTH, INC. (2020a). *FLO Period & Ovulation Tracker* (4.45.0) [Mobile Application Software]. Google Play. https://play.google.com/store/apps/details?id=org.iggymedia.periodtracker&hl=en_US

FLO HEALTH, INC. (2020b). *FLO Period & Ovulation Tracker* (iOS Version 4.59) [Mobile Application Software]. App Store. https://apps.apple.com/us/app/flo-period-tracker-ovulation/id1038369065

Fromme, J. (2003). Computer games as a part of children's culture. *Game Studies, 3*(1), 49–62.

Good Karma Applications, INC. (2020). *First-Then Visual Schedule* (iOS Version 1.1–6) [Mobile Application Software]. App store. https://apps.apple.com/us/app/first-then-visual-schedule/id355527801

Google Inc. (2020). *YouTube* (iOS Version 15.11) [Mobile Application Software]. App store. https://apps.apple.com/us/app/youtube-watch-listen-stream/id544007664

Google LLC. (2020, April 20). *Google Play Home Menu.* Google Play: https://play.google.com/store?hl=en_US

Google LLC. (2020). *YouTube* (Varies with device) [Mobile Application Software]. Google Play. https://play.google.com/store/apps/details?id=com.google.android.youtube&hl=en_US

Grande, T. (2019). Eight Signs of a Good Counselor/Therapist [Video file]. YouTube. https://www.youtube.com/watch?v=qoJBAF5q5hw

Grembe Apps Inc. (2020). *iReward* (iOS Version 4.1) [Mobile Application Software]. App store. https://apps.apple.com/us/app/ireward/id324643198

Grossman, L. (2007, January 12). The apple of your ear. *Time.* http://content.time.com/time/magazine/article/0,9171,1576854,00.html

Habitics. (2020). *Daylio Journal* (1.30.1) [Mobile Application Software]. Google Play. https://play.google.com/store/apps/details?id=net.daylio&hl=en_US

Hales, S., Turner-McGrievy, G. M., Wilcox, S., Fahim, A., Davis, R. E., Huhns, M., & Valafar, H. (2016). Social networks for improving healthy weight loss behaviors for overweight an obese adults: A randomized clinical trial of the Social Pounds Off Digitally (Social POD) mobile app. *International Journal of Medical Informatics, 94,* 81–90. https://doi.org/10.1016/j.ijmedinf.2016.07.003

Harris, S. (2020). Making Sense Podcast [Audio podcast]. https://samharris.org/podcast/

Headspace Inc. (2020a). *Headspace* (iOS Version 3.104.0) [Mobile Application Software]. App Store. https://apps.apple.com/us/app/headspace-meditation-sleep/id493145008

Headspace for Meditation, Mindfulness and Sleep. (2020b). *Headspace* (3.57.0) [Mobile Application Software]. Google Play. https://play.google.com/store/apps/details?id=com.getsomeheadspace.android&hl=en_US

HSM Studio. (2020). *Focus Keeper* (1.0.1) [Mobile Application Software]. Google Play. https://play.google.com/store/apps/details?id=com.focus_keeper&hl=en_US

IAC Search & Media Technologies Limited. (2020). *Productive* (iOS Version 2.4.0) [Mobile Application Software]. App Store. https://apps.apple.com/us/app/productive-habit-tracker/id983826477

I Am Sober LLC. (2020a). *I Am Sober* (4.8) [Mobile Application Software]. Google Play. https://play.google.com/store/apps/details?id=com.thehungrywasp.iamsober&hl=en_US

I Am Sober LLC. (2020b). *I Am Sober* (iOS Version 4.7) [Mobile Application Software]. App store. https://apps.apple.com/us/app/i-am-sober/id672904239

Influence Central. (2016). *Kids & tech: The evolution of today's digital natives.* Author. http://influence-central.com/kids-tech-the-evolution-of-todays-digital-natives/

Inozu, M., Celikcan, U., Akin, B., & Mustafaoğlu Cicek, N. (2020). The use of virtual reality (VR) exposure for reducing contamination fear and disgust: Can VR be an effective alternative exposure technique to in vivo? *Journal of Obsessive-Compulsive and Related Disorder, 25,* 1–9. https://doi.org/10.1016/j.jocrd.2020.100518

Jones, M., Dickter, B., Beard, C., Perales, R., & Bunge, E. L. (2016). Meta-analysis on cognitive behavioral treatment and behavioral intervention technologies for anxious youth: More than a BIT effective. *Contemporary Behavioral Health Care, 2*(1), 1–9. https://doi.org/10.15761/CBHC.1000115

Lenhart, A. (2015, August 6). *Teens, technology and friendships*. Pew Research Center. https://www.pewresearch.org/internet/2015/08/06/teens-technology-and-friendships/

Luden, I. (2018, January 18). Education quiz app Kahoot says it's now used by 50% of all US K-12 students, 70M users overall. *TechCrunch*. https://techcrunch.com/2018/01/18/education-quiz-app-kahoot-says-its-now-used-in-50-of-all-us-classrooms-70m-users-overall/

MapMyFitness, Inc. (2020). *MapMyFitness* (20.6.1) [Mobile Application Software]. Google Play. https://play.google.com/store/apps/details?id=com.mapmyfitness.android2&hl=en_US

Mays, D., Cremeens, J., Usdan, S., Martin, R. J., Arriola, K. J., & Bernhardt, J. M. (2010). The feasibility of assessing alcohol use among college students using wireless mobile devices: Implications for health education and behavioural research. *Health Education Journal, 69*(3), 311–320. https://doi.org/10.1177/0017896910364831

Medisafe®. (2020a). *Medisafe Medication Management* (8.76.09159) [Mobile Application Software]. Google Play. https://play.google.com/store/apps/details?id=com.medisafe.android.client&hl=en_US

Medisafe Inc. (2020b). *Medisafe Medication Management* (iOS Version 6.5.10) [Mobile Application Software]. App Store. https://apps.apple.com/us/app/medisafe-medication-management/id573916946

MHA-NYC. (2020). *My3—Support network* (5.2.0) [Mobile Application Software]. Google Play. https://play.google.com/store/apps/details?id=com.nerdery.my3&hl=en_US

Mohr, D. C., Burns, M. N., Schueller, S. M., Clarke, G., & Klinkman, M. (2013). Behavioral intervention technologies: Evidence review and recommendations for future research. *General Hospital Psychiatry, 35*(4), 332–338. https://doi.org/10.1016/j.genhosppsych.2013.03.008

MoodTools. (2020a). *Suicide Safety Plan* (iOS Version 1.4.1) [Mobile Application Software]. App store. https://apps.apple.com/us/app/suicide-safety-plan/id1003891579

MoodTools. (2020b). *Suicide Safety Plan* (1.8) [Mobile Application Software]. Google Play. https://play.google.com/store/apps/details?id=com.moodtools.crisis.app&hl=en_US

MyFitnessPal, Inc. (2020). *MyFitnessPal* (Varies with device) [Mobile Application Software]. Google Play. https://play.google.com/store/apps/details?id=com.myfitnesspal.android&hl=en_US

National Association of School Psychologists. (2019). *Shortage of school psychologists*. https://www.nasponline.org/research-and-policy/policy-priorities/critical-policy-issues/shortage-of-school-psychologists

Nguyen, T., & Davis, K. (2017). *The state of mental health in America 2017*. Mental Health America. https://www.mhanational.org/state-mental-health-america-past-reports

Oblinger, D. G. (2004). The next generation of educational engagement. *Journal of Interactive Media in Education, 2004*(1), 1–18. https://doi.org/10.5334/2004-8-oblinger

One Drop. (2020). *One Drop Diabetes Management* (2.0.30374) [Mobile Application Software]. Google Play. https://play.google.com/store/apps/details?id=today.onedrop.android&hl=en_US

One Drop and Informed Data Systems Inc. (2020). *One Drop Diabetes Management* (iOS Version 5.10.0) [Mobile Application Software]. App Store. https://apps.apple.com/us/app/one-drop-diabetes-management/id972238816

Pennant, M. E., Loucas, C. E., Whittington, C., Creswell, C., Fonagy, P., Fuggle, P., Kelvin, R., Naqvi, S., Stockton, S., & Kendall, T. (2015). Computerised therapies for anxiety and depression in children and young people: A systematic review and meta-analysis. *Behaviour Research and Therapy, 67*, 1–18. https://doi.org/10.1016/j.brat.2015.01.009

Pierce, J. M., Spriggs, A. D., Gast, D. L., & Luscre, D. (2013). Effects of visual activity schedules on independent classroom transitions for students with autism. *International Journal of Disability, Development, and Education, 60*(3), 253–269. https://doi.org/10.1080/1034912X.2013.812191

PIXO Incorporation. (2020). *Focus Keeper* (iOS Version 1.9.9) [Mobile Application Software]. App store. https://apps.apple.com/us/app/focus-keeper-time-management/id867374917

Polarised Light Ltd. (2020). *A Soft Murmur* (iOS Version 1.0.3) [Mobile Application Software]. App store. https://apps.apple.com/us/app/a-soft-murmur/id1175522255

Quizlet, Inc. (2020a). *Quizlet* (iOS Version 4.38.1) [Mobile app]. App store. https://apps.apple.com/us/app/quizlet/id546473125

Quizlet, Inc. (2020b). *Quizlet* (Varies with device) [Mobile Application Software]. Google Play. https://play.google.com/store/apps/details?id=com.quizlet.quizletandroid&hl=en_US

Raento, M., Oulasvirta, A., & Eagle, N. (2009). Smartphones: An emerging tool for social scientists. *Sociological Methods & Research, 37*(2), 426–454. https://doi.org/10.1177/0049124108330005

Rapoff, M. A. (2010). *Adherence to pediatric medical regimens* (2nd ed.). Springer US. https://doi.org/10.1007/978-1-4419-0570-3

Relaxio. (2020). *Daylio Journal* (iOS Version 1.19.4) [Mobile Application Software]. App Store. https://apps.apple.com/us/app/daylio-journal/id1194023242

Rideout, V., & Robb, M. B. (2019). *The Common Sense census: Media use by tweens and teens, 2019*. Common Sense Media.

Silang, J. P. (2020). *Study Bunny* (iOS Version 15.0.9) [Mobile Application Software]. App store. https://apps.apple.com/tm/app/study-bunny-focus-timer/id1478345385

Sleepy Rabbit LLC. (2020). *A Soft Murmur* (2.1.1) [Mobile Application Software]. Google Play. https://play.google.com/store/apps/details?id=com.gabemart.asoftmurmur&hl=en_US

Smillage, Inc. (2020). *Step Younger+* (iOS Version 1.1.9) [Mobile Application Software]. App Store. https://apps.apple.com/us/app/step-younger/id1494267894

SoberTool. (2020). *SoberTool* (6.0.1-lite) [Mobile Application Software]. Google Play. https://play.google.com/store/apps/details?id=com.osu.cleanandsobertoolboxandroid&hl=en_US

Sormunen, M., & Miettinen, H. (2017). Health behavior tracking via mobile games: A case study among school-aged children. *Cogent Education, 4*, 1–11. https://doi.org/10.1080/2331186X.2017.1311500

Spotify Ltd. (2020a). *Spotify* (iOS Version 8.5.49) [Mobile Application Software]. Mobile app. https://apps.apple.com/us/app/spotify-music-and-podcasts/id324684580

Spotify Ltd. (2020b). *Spotify* (Varies with device) [Mobile Application Software]. Google Play. https://play.google.com/store/apps/details?id=com.spotify.music&hl=en_US

Sugie, N. F. (2018). Utilizing smartphones to study disadvantaged and hard-to-reach groups. *Sociological Methods & Research, 47*(3), 458–491. doi:10.1177/0049124115626176

SuperByte. (2020). *Study Bunny* (15.1.1) [Mobile Application Software]. Google Play. https://play.google.com/store/apps/details?id=com.superbyte.studybunny&hl=en_US

Time Timer, LLC. (2020a). *Time Timer* (iOS Version 3.3.6) [Mobile Application Software]. App store. https://apps.apple.com/us/app/time-timer/id332520417

Time Timer, LLC. (2020b). *Time Timer* (3.0.3 b1024) [Mobile Application Software]. Google Play. https://play.google.com/store/apps/details?id=com.timetimer.android&hl=en_US

Tompkins, M. A., & Martinez, K. A. (2010). *My anxious mind: A teen's guide to managing anxiety and panic*. Sheridan Books.

Trevor Project. (2020). https://www.thetrevorproject.org/

Under Armour Inc. (2020a). *MapMyFitness* (iOS Version 1.3.5) [Mobile Application Software]. App Store. https://apps.apple.com/us/app/map-my-fitness-by-under-armour/id298903147

Under Armour, Inc. (2020b). *MyFitnessPal* (iOS Version 20.5.0) [Mobile Application Software]. App Store. https://apps.apple.com/us/app/myfitnesspal/id341232718

University of Wolongong. (2019, March 22). *Understanding operating systems*. https://www.uow.edu.au/student/learning-co-op/technology-and-software/operating-systems

Urech, A., Krieger, T., Chesham, A., Mast, F. W., & Berger, T. (2015). Virtual reality-based attention bias modification training for social anxiety: A feasibility and proof of concept study. *Frontiers in Psychiatry, 6*, 1–5. https://doi.org/10.3389/fpsyt.2015.00154

Waking Up LLC. (2020a). *Waking Up: A Meditation Course* (iOS Version 1.3.94) [Mobile Application Software]. App Store. https://apps.apple.com/us/app/waking-up-a-meditation-course/id1307736395

Waking Up LLC. (2020b). *Waking Up: A Meditation Course* (1.5.4) [Mobile Application Software]. Google Play. https://play.google.com/store/apps/details?id=org.wakingup.android&hl=en_US

Whitney, D. G., & Peterson, M. D. (2019). US national and state-level prevalence of mental health disorders and disparities of mental health care use in children. *JAMA Pediatrics, 173*(4), 389–391. https://doi.org 10.1001/jamapediatrics.2018.5399

Winslow, B. D., Chadderdon, G. L., Dechmerowski, S. J., Jones, D. L., Kalkstein, S., Greene, J. L., & Gehrman, P. (2016). Development and clinical evaluation of an mHealth application for stress management. *Frontiers in Psychiatry, 7*, 1–8. https://doi.org/10.3389/fpsyt.2016.00130

World Health Organization. (2019, October 23). *Adolescent mental health fact sheet*. https://www.who.int/news-room/fact-sheets/detail/adolescent-mental-health

Zidani, M., Audet, J.-S., Borgeat, F., Aardema, F., O'Connor, K. P., & Khazzal, Y. (2017). Augmentation of psychotherapy through alternative preconscious priming: A case series exploring effects on residual symptoms. *Frontiers in Psychiatry, 8*, 1–6. https://doi.org/10.3389/fpsyt.2017.00008

9

Terminating Therapy and Referrals

JASON GALLANT, DIANA JOYCE-BEAULIEU, AND BRIAN A. ZABOSKI ■

The decision to terminate therapy often follows when a client's goals have been met and the individual is ready to function independently. This is the closure circumstance that counselors and clients hope for. However, in some cases, an interruption of services or termination of therapy may be due to personal circumstances (e.g., military deployment, relocation, illness) of the therapist or client. More problematic conditions such as significant absenteeism from appointments, intervention refusal, an ineffective client/counselor match, or lack of progress also may be causes for termination of therapy. Regardless of the precipitating situation, good planning for closure offers an important final opportunity to support the student.

PREPARATION FOR CLOSURE

Transition planning, booster sessions, and at times referrals to other providers can provide closure to the therapeutic relationship. Transition planning begins with a review of the client's goals, progress toward those goals, and assessment of their current functioning. There also are ethical guidelines on interruption or termination of services across several national professional organizations (e.g., American Psychological Association [APA], National Association of School Psychologists [NASP], American Counseling Association [ACA], and National Association of Social Workers [NASW]). As an example, the APA's *Ethical Principles of Psychologists and Code of Conduct* provisions discuss interruption of services that might occur (e.g., a therapist changes employment contracts or retires; a client fails to benefit from therapy; APA, 2017). The overarching principle strongly considers the client's well-being and includes the following three provisions:

(a) Psychologists terminate therapy when it becomes reasonably clear that the client/patient no longer needs the service, is not likely to benefit, or is being harmed by continued service.
(b) Psychologists may terminate therapy when threatened or otherwise endangered by the client/patient or another person with whom the client/patient has a relationship.
(c) Except where precluded by the actions of clients/patients or third-party payers, prior to termination psychologists provide pretermination counseling and suggest alternative service providers as appropriate. (APA, 2017, section 10.09)

If a counselor determines that therapy goals have been successful, progress data indicate a stable pattern of improvement, and the client is no longer functionally impaired, there is usually justification to withdraw the intervention. Even in the best-case scenarios, mental health professionals understand that human emotional functioning and behaviors can fluctuate over time, especially when stressors arise or new challenges are presented. Therefore, ensuring that the client has a plan to address unforeseen future setbacks is a good strategy. Simple steps in transition planning may include the following:

(a) Giving advance notice of the upcoming final sessions can help clients acclimate to the change. This is especially important when personal attachment or the therapeutic alliance has been strong or the client has experienced abandonment in past relationships.
(b) Reviewing strategies learned and answering any lingering questions can help solidify the knowledge gained in counseling.
(c) Discussing contingency plans if stressors should arise can also facilitate future success. This might take the form of practice scenarios, role plays, or just brainstorming options (e.g., "What are some strategies you learned that you can use if you start to feel anxious prior to your exams?").
(d) Ensuring that the client can access a variety of resources (e.g., online support groups, contact info for counselors, checklists of strategies that worked for the individual, contact info for a sponsor, a "go-to" adult, and perhaps crisis hotline numbers) during the transition period.
(e) For those clients who are moving to other locations, it will be important to make sure they are aware of resources in the new location. For example, graduating high school students may benefit from knowing that colleges have student mental health centers and that employers typically offer Employee Assistance Programs that provide several free counseling sessions, should those be needed. Students who have enlisted may need awareness of support systems within the military, and those who are being adjudicated may need information on how to quickly connect with mental health supports within the juvenile justice system

(e.g., this can be requested during the intake session when they arrive at the facility).
(f) Celebrating goals attained throughout the therapy can provide a form of empowerment.
(g) Lastly, it is important for therapists to summarize their clinical notes and ensure there is a mechanism to share those with the client or next provider, if requested.

When transition plans are prompted by absenteeism, refusal of services, or ineffective match between the client and therapist, there also are additional options. For absenteeism, a clinical interview that tries to understand and remove the barriers to attendance is the first step. As an example, a child who is undergoing intensive chemotherapy treatments may be unable to attend for several months. Thus, the transition meeting can include a discussion of temporary resources offered by hospital rehabilitation professionals, family support groups, and a reentry plan for the child once treatment is completed. For students who refuse to participate in counseling, incentive plans may be helpful, a temporary hiatus may be beneficial, or at times a different therapist might be a better match (e.g., a teenage boy may prefer a male therapist). There also are circumstances where therapists may feel endangered by a client, so a referral to a therapist specializing in conduct disorders or antisocial behaviors may be appropriate. When therapy rapport and techniques have been strong yet there is little progress, referrals to outside care providers (e.g., psychiatrist, pediatrician) for a medical consultation or family therapy may be included within transition planning. Referrals and collaboration with outside providers are discussed in more detail at the end of this chapter.

BOOSTER SESSIONS

The term "booster sessions" refers to one or more additional therapy meetings offered after the core therapy sequence has been completed. The purpose is to check on progress, review strategies learned during therapy, answer any new questions, and provide additional temporary supports or resources if needed. Booster sessions focus on the applied aspects of the techniques that were taught (e.g., "Is the client generalizing the strategies outside of the therapy room and using them correctly?," "Are the strategies successful?," "Are there any skill gaps that need to be reviewed?"). The boosters are not intended to introduce new material or curricula. For some students the booster serves to solidify concepts they learned and offers an opportunity for the therapist to validate their progress. Typically, the booster occurs after a month or longer has elapsed and may be just one session or a series of sessions (e.g., monthly or by semester). In school systems, the booster might occur at natural progress-monitoring points following completion of therapy (e.g., monthly, end of quarter) or following transition points such as the beginning of a new semester or after significant breaks (e.g., winter holidays, spring break, summer vacation).

There is significant literature supporting the effectiveness of this technique for sustaining counseling progress across ages and presenting problems. In a study of 94 pediatric patients with obsessive-compulsive disorder (OCD) receiving 12 weeks of family-based cognitive behavioral therapy (CBT), researchers offered an option for drop-in booster sessions over 6-months (Negreiros et al., 2019). They found that most families accessed the booster sessions (mean of 2.84 sessions attended) and reported benefits for peer interactions, feeling supported, skill reviews, and homework development. Parents of children with comorbidities were more likely to attend and participate than those whose child only had OCD (82% and 58% respectively). A separate study of 123 adolescents with depression found that adding booster sessions (every 4 months for 24 months) to a CBT program accelerated the recovery from depression compared to those who did not receive booster sessions (Clarke et al., 1999). However, it did not reduce the recurrence rate of additional depression episodes between groups.

In a meta-analysis of 53 CBT studies for anxiety and mood disorders, researchers found significantly larger effect sizes for studies with booster sessions ($r = 0.58$) compared to those without booster sessions ($r = 0.45$; Gearing et al., 2013). CBT coupled with booster sessions has also been found to have significant positive results when addressing binge eating disorder. In their study of 36 females, Schlup et al. (2009) provided eight weekly sessions of CBT to all participants and then either five 90-minute booster sessions over a year or a waitlist condition. Follow-up measurement was taken at 12 months. Individuals receiving the CBT with booster sessions had significantly fewer binge eating episodes than those in the control condition, although the control group also had a small reduction in binge eating episodes. The percentage of females who abstained from any binge eating rose from 0% to 39% in the treatment group but remained at 0% for the control group at 12 months after treatment.

REFERRALS FOR EXTENDED OR MULTIFACETED CARE

Collaboration and coordination of services with external mental health providers are often required when youth have multifaceted, complex mental health needs (Stancin & Perrin, 2014). Given their knowledge of child development, school services infrastructure, and the broader medical community, school psychologists can serve as a liaison and resource for families necessitating follow-up treatment. Numerous options are available to families in bridging school-based and outpatient treatment, and these options may be conceptualized as a continuum of services from least to most intensive. Possible external mental health options may include community youth programs, outpatient mental health clinic services, in-home family services, intensive treatment centers, inpatient hospitalization, and residential placements, as well as psychopharmacology.

Treatment options may be provided simultaneously, and access to one or numerous modalities is contingent on symptom severity and assessed needs. Therefore, conducting a suitable needs assessment is an essential first step for school psychologists to ensure that the family initiates care at the most appropriate and least restrictive service level. Prior to seeking an external mental health treatment option, the school psychologist should consider numerous factors that enhance suitability of fit, eliminate confusion about the mental health treatment process, and increase probability of adherence (Nock & Ferriter, 2005). In fact, school psychologists are well equipped to perform a needs assessment as they have access to years of information about school performance, intervention response, and behavioral patterns; opportunities for in vivo observations; contact with raters across settings; and parents' input on developmental history. Determining the appropriate level of services and locating a suitable provider can present as a daunting undertaking for families. Confused or overwhelmed families may fail to initiate important services; thus, the school psychologist's referral can guide families to outside providers and encourage them to seek help (Brown et al., 2014).

FACTORS IMPACTING TREATMENT ENGAGEMENT

Because approximately 20% to 60% of families who contact do not attend ("no-show") their initial appointment, practitioners should understand the many barriers that interfere with treatment (Benway et al., 2003; Pellerin et al., 2010). These factors can be divided into two types. *Pragmatic factors* include financial challenges, distance, wait time, and lack of transportation, while *perceived challenges* encompass negative experiences and stigma regarding service utilization (Bannon & McKay, 2005; Reardon et al., 2017; Sherman et al., 2008; Swift et al., 2012).

Pragmatic Challenges

Financial considerations pervasively impact treatment engagement; therefore, it is helpful for practitioners to understand insurance and payment options to convey accurate information to families (Reardon et al., 2017). Three common payment options are available to families seeking outpatient mental health services: private insurance, public insurance, and private pay.

The cost that families incur when using private insurance depends on their provider and insurance policy. Private insurance companies vary by state, but some of the most common national insurance plans are United Healthcare, Blue Cross Blue Shield, Aetna, and Cigna. When mental health providers seek inclusion with one of these private insurance companies the process is called "paneling" or "credentialing." Once the clinician is accepted onto the insurance it is called "being credentialed" or "being paneled," which enters them into a contractual agreement with the insurance company. The insurance company will then dictate the rate per service, and the mental health provider will have the option to accept or deny that rate. When a family arrives for treatment, they will be required to pay their portion of the contracted rate as dictated by their insurance policy.

Consider an example where a psychologist is credentialed with United Healthcare and agreed to accept a rate of $100 per individual and family therapy session. Each time the provider sees a family and bills for the service, United Healthcare will pay a total of $100. The Smith family has a co-pay of $40 as indicated by their insurance policy. Thus, when they arrive to treatment the Smith family will pay $40. After the session, the provider will bill the insurance company for the remainder of the agreement. The provider should receive $60 from the insurance company.

In other situations, families have a deductible plan. With the deductible plan, families pay the full rate of service until they meet a certain level of out-of-pocket expense. (The threshold of these out-of-pocket expenses varies depending on the plan.) In the previous example, a family who has not met their yearly deductible would have to pay the full $100 rate. Once the family meets their out-of-pocket expenses, in most cases, they would then owe $0 and the insurance company would pay the full contractual rate for the remainder of the calendar year. The deductible resets at the beginning of each calendar year.

Families with private insurance will often seek mental health providers who are on their insurance panel given that the co-pay or deductible is traditionally cheaper than private-pay rates. Almost all insurance companies have a provider search portal. It may be beneficial for school psychologists to share this information with families to help them navigate the provider search process.

Public insurance (e.g., Medicaid and Children's Health Insurance Program) is a national public health program for families with low income. Approximately 20% of Americans are covered by Medicaid (Rudowitz & Garfield, 2019). Public health programs like Medicaid cover approximately 83% of children in poverty and 48% of children with unique health needs (i.e., chronic physical, developmental, behavioral, or mental health risk). Public insurance eligibility varies by state: The 48 contiguous states cover children with family incomes at or above 200% of the Federal Poverty Level ($43,440 per year for a family of three in 2020). Alaska and Hawaii include a higher income range for eligibility ($65,160 per year for a family of three in 2020) (U.S. Department of Health and Human Services, 2020). The paneling process is similar to that in private insurance. In many states, youth with Medicaid receive free mental health services, with possible limitations on the frequency and number of sessions per calendar year. Traditionally, Medicaid reimburses providers less than private insurance and private-pay rates (Cohn & Hastings, 2013). In lieu of lower reimbursement rates and challenges with treatment attendance (Guck et al., 2007), providers may be less inclined to seek Medicaid paneling. Therefore, school districts might consider building relationships with local community mental health centers, institutions, and nonprofit organizations who serve families on public insurance.

Nonprofits and community mental health centers may offer free or low-cost services (i.e., in-home family services [IHFS]) paid by local contracts and grants.

In addition, pastoral (e.g., Catholic Charities) and self-help groups counseling (e.g., Teen Alcohol Rehab, Al-Anon for families of alcoholics, and Nar-Anon for families with drug addictions) may be offered for free or for a small sliding-scale fee. Sliding-scale payments are adjusted based on the individual's income level, so the lower the income, the lower the session payment required. However, suitability of free treatment for kids and families must be carefully reviewed, and it is important to be sensitive to family preferences regarding faith-based services. Overall, by establishing relationships with community agencies, nonprofit organizations, and religious institutions, the school psychologist can stay current on local programs and services available to families regardless of their insurance coverage. School systems generally do not recommend specific providers but may provide a list of local resource options.

Families seeking private-pay options either do not have insurance coverage or want to work with a specific provider outside their insurance network. Families may elect for private pay to avoid long wait times for appointments or to seek specialized expertise. Private-pay rates vary by geographic region and the provider's expertise and may be prohibitive for many families. In building a relationship with private-pay providers, school districts can document typical length of treatment and services offered. High quality, specialized expertise, and timely service delivery are particularly important to families paying privately.

Logistic and financial barriers (other than payment) may also influence treatment engagement—for example, missed work and transportation costs (i.e., gas and tolls; Salloum et al., 2016). In addition, treatment facilities and practices with long wait times may inhibit treatment attendance (Ofonedu et al., 2017; Sherman et al., 2008; Swift et al., 2012). Numerous other factors like scheduling for extracurricular hobbies (e.g., soccer, ballet, Scouts), household composition, and single-parent status may uniquely impact the probability of family involvement. Thus, educating families on distance, costs, and wait times can augment treatment engagement. For instance, consider a single parent who works an hourly job. This parent may be limited to attending appointments after work, meaning they will likely be driving during rush hour, which will lengthen the travel time and lead to higher gas costs, which ultimately decreases the probability of attendance. Additionally, outside providers usually have attendance policies: Families who miss appointments can be dropped from the patient list. This is particularly pertinent for (a) specialty providers with long waitlists or (b) more intensive treatment that insurance companies may stop paying for due to high absenteeism. Assessing for logistical and pragmatic barriers should be an essential component of external referrals.

Perceived Challenges

Views and perceptions about the therapeutic experience are also commonly tied to treatment engagement. Research has shown that engagement is impacted by hoping for positive outcomes (Constantino et al., 2011; Swift et al., 2012), positive attitudes toward psychological treatment (Gonzalez et al., 2002; Swift & Callahan, 2010), trust in mental health professionals (Ofonedu et al., 2017), lack of education about the mental health treatment process (Brown et al., 2014), and the fear of stigma or blame (Dempster et al., 2015). The school psychologist should consider meeting with families prior to the external referral to assess these factors. The brief interaction could include questions about a parent's knowledge and views of CBT, their understanding of the outpatient treatment process, past treatment utilization experiences, and any fears they may have about mental health services. In doing so, the school psychologist has the opportunity to dispel those concerns and thus may increase attendance outside of school-based care (Brown et al., 2014).

TREATMENT OPTIONS

Outpatient Mental Health Services

Outpatient mental health services consist of treatment administered at a clinic or facility. Sessions are typically scheduled on a weekly, biweekly, or monthly basis and last approximately 30 minutes to 1 hour. Treatment duration is contingent on numerous factors, including symptom presentation, symptom severity, treatment philosophy, and intervention adherence. Outpatient services can be further broken down into primary, traditional, and specialty care.

PRIMARY CARE PEDIATRIC PSYCHOLOGY

Primary care pediatric psychology emphasizes early intervention through the establishment of sound relationships with pediatricians (Friman, 2010). Pediatricians are particularly helpful colleagues as they have regular interactions with youth and their parents. However, pediatricians report lower confidence with social-emotional problems (Stein et al., 2008), even though 60% of all annual pediatric well-check visits include some kind of behavioral concern (Arndorfer et al., 1999). Thus, psychologists and pediatricians can collaborate to facilitate early detection of emotional and behavioral difficulties. Indeed, early intervention has beneficial outcomes across childhood development (Wolk et al., 2015). Consider a 4-year-old who frequently and defiantly says "No, mommy!" to requests. Difficulties accepting decisions and following instructions are cardinal issues in early childhood. Nevertheless, without adequate parenting tools, "No, mommy!" at age 4 may turn into much more significant and challenging oppositional behaviors in the teenage years.

Primary care pediatric psychologists can be viewed as the pediatricians of the mental health world. Generalists by nature, these providers have a wealth of competencies to treat common concerns early in their manifestation. Primary care pediatric psychologists specialize in the treatment of common behavioral and psychological problems such as anxiety, mood concerns, academic struggles, sleep difficulties, picky eating, sibling conflicts, frustration tolerance, and emotional coping issues. Primary care psychologists typically understand child behavior from an external, contextual, and circumstantial framework. That is, child behavior is not so much a reflection of internal deficits or psychological flaws as it is a reflection of the context not meeting the child's needs. This concept can be further illustrated in the "banana tree" metaphor. A banana tree thrives in tropical climates with an abundance of precipitation, warm weather, and fertilizer. If you took that banana tree and placed it in the middle of the desert, it would not have the resources needed to thrive and survive. Now does that mean that the banana tree is deficient? Not exactly. Does that suggest that the desert is a bad environment? Not necessarily. It is the mismatch between the banana tree's needs and what the desert offers that presents a challenge.

Given the perspective that contextual factors are the culprit in early child behavioral problems, treatment emphasizes environmental changes through parent training. Research suggests that parent training improves the therapeutic experience above and beyond child-focused treatment (Dowell & Ogles, 2010). Within a primary care perspective, parent-focused treatment has two chief components: targeted health education and prescriptive behavioral treatments (Friman, 2010). Targeted health education focuses on teaching parents about typical behavioral problems and about health-related behaviors that may impact functioning (e.g., telling parents about the necessary hours of sleep per night for a child or helping them to understand that having imaginary friends is a normal part of early childhood). Prescriptive behavioral treatments consist of specific steps necessary for achieving goals. A parent who wants their child to remain in their own bed at night may benefit from a step-by-step "prescription" on how to ensure independent sleep and prevent co-sleeping. Overall, primary care pediatric psychologists can serve as a valuable resource for children and families seeking services before problems turn into more significant pathology. Thus, school psychologists should be aware of these providers and convey that information through family consultation.

Traditional Child Psychotherapy

Traditional child mental health treatment is a broad umbrella term that may suggest a myriad of intervention strategies and perspectives. One estimate suggested there were approximately 551 different therapeutic strategies used with children and adolescents (Kazdin, 2000; Weisz & Kazdin, 2018). For instance, a provider may use elements of play therapy to build rapport, cognitive therapy to restructure negative thoughts, and parent training for behavioral concerns at home. Ultimately, school psychologists must know their referral sources and follow up with families to understand the type of therapy they receive and the goals of that intervention.

Specialty Care

Specialty-level services are administered by providers who focus on a particular diagnosis or presenting problem. These providers may practice exclusively with children with OCD, tic disorders, or anxiety disorders; alternatively, they may focus on specific groups like children experiencing grief or victims of sexual abuse.

Adjunct therapies could also meet criteria for specialty-level services. Adjunct therapies are considered supplemental to individual therapy rather than a replacement. Some examples include biofeedback for posttraumatic stress disorder, a grief support group, or a social skills group. The school psychologist should consider child/family needs, treatment preferences, empirical support, and suitability for the family when making referrals for adjunct treatments. Remember, the child's pediatrician may also have extensive knowledge of and experiences with outpatient mental health providers in a given geographic region. Using their knowledge of quality providers could be an asset to the child and family.

In-Home Family Services

IHFS is an omnibus term for an array of therapeutic services administered in a child's home (Ingram et al., 2015). In-home services are a valuable element of care for families with difficulties accessing services in a traditional office format. They can be quite versatile and used for a range of presenting problems and functions, including families referred by child welfare agencies due to difficulty providing a stable home environment (Batenhorst et al., 2011). Like outpatient clinics, providers working in IHFS programs assess for deficits, administer skills-based interventions, and generalize skills to other environments (Batenhorst et al., 2011). As an example, IHFS may help scaffold parenting skills by teaching parents strategies to use in the home, assisting them in understanding their own histories of abuse, and suggesting ways to change those patterns. IHFS can also benefit youth who are reuniting with their family after completing a higher level of care (e.g., residential), have failed to respond to traditional outpatient therapy, present with challenges accessing traditional outpatient therapy, are at risk for removal from the home, experience school problems, or require applied behavioral analysis (Hurley et al., 2011; Reed et al., 2007; Spielberger et al., 2010). The frequency and the duration of IHFS vary according to the referral concern and the severity of presenting symptoms.

The education and training of an IHFS provider differ by the company or organization. These services could be administered by a licensed psychologist, a master's-level board-certified behavioral analyst, a licensed counselor, or a bachelor's-level behavioral consultant. School-based clinicians should be aware of IHFS offered in their area. Contacting companies and organizations is a reasonable way to understand their theoretical orientation, educational requirements, frequency and duration of service, and cost. Cost can vary greatly by geographic region and organization. As an example, the Boys Town Central Florida IHFS program in Orlando offers free IHFS to residents in specific counties through a local grant (Batenhorst et al., 2011). The grant dictates that services are conducted weekly for a total of 12 weeks and treatment will be administered by trained behavioral consultants at the bachelor's or master's level. Such services may also be administered as an out-of-pocket expense, while specialized applied behavior analysis services may be covered by some insurance companies. Given the subtleties in the Boys Town example, as one might imagine, simply recommending IHFS without additional guidance could be overwhelming.

Intensive Treatment

Five primary models of intensive treatment can assist youth presenting with severe emotional and behavioral problems: intensive outpatient programs (IOPs), partial hospitalization programs (PHPs), respite care, residential treatment, and inpatient hospitalization. The primary differences between each program typically consist of the frequency and duration of treatment and patient supervision.

IOPs typically consist of two to five sessions per week that last approximately 2 to 3 hours each. IOPs may be administered in a hospital or an office-like setting. Sessions can be conducted in an individual or group format and have been found to be effective for an array of presenting problems that include depression, suicidal behaviors, eating disorders, anxiety/OCD, substance abuse, and behavioral concerns (Dalle Grave et al., 2008; Kennard et al., 2019; Lewin et al., 2005; Osgood-Hynes et al., 2003; Ritschel et al., 2012).

PHPs address similar concerns but are one step up from IOPs in terms of treatment intensity. Many PHPs require attendance of 5 to 7 days a week for 4 to 6 hours per day, though patients continue to live at home (Hayes et al., 2019). PHPs often serve as a last resort before a patient stays at a residential or inpatient setting. PHPs may also use a multimodal treatment modality that includes therapy, groups, and medication management.

Respite care or emergency shelter care consists of a short-term out-of-home placement for youth who have extreme behavioral or emotional concerns, who are runaways awaiting reunification with their family, or who require temporary placement as they await a more suitable setting (Leon et al., 2016). A typical respite stay may last anywhere from 2 to 4 weeks. Shelters may serve multiple purposes: They may provide temporary respite for children with significant emotional and behavioral problems or short-term placement for children entering the child welfare system requiring residential placement. Despite widespread use, only limited empirical evidence supports the effectiveness of shelter placement (Hindt et al., 2019; Strijker et al., 2008). In a longitudinal study of 282 youth, 37% of whom had been placed in shelters, researchers found long-term elevated internalizing trajectories (i.e., depression, anxiety, and somatization) among those placed in shelters. The negative impact was somewhat attenuated for those who had visitation and continued kinship. Findings suggested that keeping youth connected in some form with their families and social networks may serve as a protective factor (Hindt et al., 2019).

The most intense intervention option is a residential program where youth live at a facility to receive daily intervention. They may be referred to residential programs by practitioners, families, judges, or caseworkers. Youth entering residential programs vary greatly. Some have been adjudicated and are being placed by a judge; others may be highly disruptive in the home and require more structure; and some may be so functionally impaired by depression or anxiety that they cannot function safely absent professional supervision.

Residential programs vary; however, they commonly mimic a highly structured home environment by requiring patients to engage in activities of daily living, adhere to mealtimes, and follow daily activity schedules. Some programs even have a married couple living with the youth to replicate a home context (Larzelere et al., 2004). They offer multimodal treatment including integration of behavioral, counseling, and psychopharmacological solutions and sometimes also have staged treatment (e.g., inpatient, intensive outpatient, transitional housing). There are a number of intensive CBT residential centers for severe psychiatric disorders throughout the country (e.g., McLean Hospital, https://www.mcleanhospital.org/ ; Silver Hill Hospital, https://silverhillhospital.org/).

The length of stay in a residential treatment program depends on several factors. For example, an adolescent with suicidal behaviors and depression may have significant improvement in a few weeks, whereas a 16-year-old undergoing drug rehabilitation with extreme and dangerous behavioral problems may stay for a year or longer. One study of 42 youth in a residential treatment program found that the length of stay ranged from 18 to 505 days, with a mean duration of 181 days (Larzelere et al., 2004).

Acute inpatient hospitalization is the most restrictive form of treatment. Inpatient hospitalization is for the most severe and unsafe behaviors (e.g., suicidal, highly aggressive, homicidal; Rice et al., 2002). Youth entering inpatient hospitalization are monitored 24 hours, 7 days a week for their own safety. Those admitted at this level of care may present with severe outbursts, may be a danger to themselves or others, and are unable to remain safe without constant supervision. While residential treatment facilities have long-term therapeutic goals, the goal of inpatient hospitalization is typically stabilization. That is, they temporarily relieve the most severe symptoms (e.g., suicidality)—especially through medication management—so that a patient can return to a less restrictive setting. As youth generally stay in inpatient units until they are no longer a danger to themselves or others, intervention duration is variable.

What If Medication Is an Option?

Many times youth present with symptoms that warrant pharmacotherapy. While some states prohibit school personnel from making medication requirements or suggestions, other states allow doctoral-level licensed psychologists to prescribe, usually with additional training. Because many of us have limited training in medication management, a comprehensive discussion is outside of the scope of this chapter. Nevertheless, for consultative and intervention-support purposes, we believe that school psychologists should at least be aware of common psychiatric medications and their side effects. An easy online reference for medications and their side effects is available at www.pdr.net (Prescriber's Digital Reference, 2020).

When medicinal interventions for an emotional, behavioral, or academic concern have been initiated by parents/guardians, there are several ways school personnel may be of assistance. First and foremost, ask the caregiver for consent to coordinate care with the child's primary care provider or pediatrician. Remember, pediatricians often have years of experience working with the family. Second, if the child is eligible for special education services and has an Individualized Education Program (IEP), medication administration may need to be incorporated into the school day. Counseling Association Lastly, school personnel can communicate with the prescribing physician about counseling and support strategies so everyone uses similar intervention techniques and language.

CHAPTER DISCUSSION QUESTIONS

1. What are the three provisions of section 10.09 of the APA's *Ethical Principles of Psychologists and Code of Conduct* regarding termination of counseling?
2. Name five key steps to ensure good transition planning for students/clients.
3. What support does the research offer for booster sessions following completion of CBT?
4. What are some of the factors and barriers that lower counseling appointment attendance for families?
5. What are some of the benefits and challenges for IHFS?
6. Compare and contrast primary care pediatric psychology, traditional child psychotherapy, inpatient, emergency shelter, and residential care options.
7. What therapist and student/client circumstances might precipitate terminating therapy?

REFERENCES

American Psychological Association. (2017). *Ethical principles of psychologists and code of conduct: Including 2010 and 2016 amendments.* https://www.apa.org/ethics/code/

Arndorfer, R. E., Allen, K. D., & Aljazireh, L. (1999). Behavioral health needs in pediatric medicine and the acceptability of behavioral solutions: Implications for behavioral psychologists. *Behavior Therapy, 30*(1), 137–148. https://doi.org/10.1016/S0005-7894(99)80050-1

Bannon, W. M., & McKay, M. M. (2005). Are barriers to service and parental preference match for service related to urban child mental health service use? *Families in Society: The Journal of Contemporary Social Services, 86*(1), 30–34. https://doi.org/10.1606/1044-3894.1874

Batenhorst, L., Simpson, A., & Thompson, R. (2011). *Boys Town in-home family services manual*. Boys Town.

Benway, C. B., Hamrin, V., & McMahon, T. J. (2003). Initial appointment nonattendance in child and family mental health clinics. *American Journal of Orthopsychiatry*, 73(4), 419–428. https://doi.org/10.1037/0002-9432.73.4.419

Brown, J. S. L., Ferner, H., Wingrove, J., Aschan, L., Hatch, S. L., & Hotopf, M. (2014). How equitable are psychological therapy services in South East London now? A comparison of referrals to a new psychological therapy service with participants in a psychiatric morbidity survey in the same London borough. *Social Psychiatry and Psychiatric Epidemiology*, 49(12), 1893–1902. https://doi.org/10.1007/s00127-014-0900-6

Clarke, G. N., Rohde, P., Lewinsohn, P. M., Hops, H., & Seeley, J. R. (1999). Cognitive-behavioral treatment of adolescent depression: Efficacy of acute group treatment and booster sessions. *Journal of the American Academy of Child & Adolescent Psychiatry*, 38(3), 272–279. https://doi.org/10.1097/00004583-199903000-00014

Cohn, T., & Hastings, S. (2013). Building a practice in rural settings: Special considerations. *Journal of Mental Health Counseling*, 35(3), 228–244. https://doi.org/10.17744/mehc.35.3.12171572424wxhll

Constantino, M. J., Arnkoff, D. B., Glass, C. R., Ametrano, R. M., & Smith, J. Z. (2011). Expectations. *Journal of Clinical Psychology*, 67(2), 184–192. https://doi.org/10.1002/jclp.20754

Dalle Grave, R., Pasqualoni, E., & Calugi, S. (2008). Intensive outpatient cognitive behaviour therapy for eating disorder. *Psihologijske Teme*, 17(2), 313–327.

Dempster, R., Davis, D. W., Faye Jones, V., Keating, A., & Wildman, B. (2015). The role of stigma in parental help-seeking for perceived child behavior problems in urban, low-income African American parents. *Journal of Clinical Psychology in Medical Settings*, 22(4), 265–278. https://doi.org/10.1007/s10880-015-9433-8

Dowell, K. A., & Ogles, B. M. (2010). The effects of parent participation on child psychotherapy outcome: A meta-analytic review. *Journal of Clinical Child & Adolescent Psychology*, 39(2), 151–162. https://doi.org/10.1080/15374410903532585

Friman, P. C. (2010). Come on in, the water is fine: Achieving mainstream relevance through integration with primary medical care. *Behavior Analyst*, 33(1), 19–36. https://doi.org/10.1007/BF03392201

Gearing, R. E., Schwalbe, C. S., Lee, R. H., & Hoagwood, K. E. (2013). The effectiveness of booster sessions in CBT treatment for child and adolescent mood and anxiety disorders. *Depression & Anxiety*, 30(9), 800–808. https://doi.org/10.1002/da.22118

Gonzalez, J. M., Tinsley, H. E. A., & Kreuder, K. R. (2002). Effects of psychoeducational interventions on opinions of mental illness, attitudes toward help seeking, and expectations about psychotherapy in college students. *Journal of College Student Development*, 43(1), 51–63.

Guck, T. P., Guck, A. J., Brack, A. B., & Frey, D. R. (2007). No-show rates in partially integrated models of behavioral health care in a primary care setting. *Families, Systems, & Health*, 25(2), 137–146. https://doi.org/10.1037/1091-7527.25.2.137

Hayes, N. A., Welty, L. J., Slesinger, N., & Washburn, J. J. (2019). Moderators of treatment outcomes in a partial hospitalization and intensive outpatient program for eating disorders. *Eating Disorders*, 27(3), 305–320. https://doi.org/10.1080/10640266.2018.1512302

Hindt, L. A., Jhe Bai, G., Huguenel, B. M., Fuller, A. K., & Leon, S. C. (2019). Impact of emergency shelter utilization and kinship involvement on children's behavioral outcomes. *Child Maltreatment, 24*(1), 76–85. https://doi.org/10.1177/1077559518797198

Hurley, K. D., Griffith, A. L., Casey, K., Ingram, S., & Simpson, A. (2011). Behavioral and emotional outcomes of an in-home parent training intervention for young children. *Journal of At-Risk Issues, 16*(2), 1–7.

Ingram, S. D., Cash, S. J., Oats, R. G., Simpson, A., & Thompson, R. W. (2015). Development of an evidence-informed in-home family services model for families and children at risk of abuse and neglect: Evidence-informed in-home family services model. *Child & Family Social Work, 20*(2), 139–148. https://doi.org/10.1111/cfs.12061

Kazdin, A. E. (2000). *Psychotherapy for children and adolescents: Directions for research and practice*. Oxford University Press.

Kennard, B., Mayes, T., King, J., Moorehead, A., Wolfe, K., Hughes, J., Castillo, B., Smith, M., Matney, J., Oscarson, B., Stewart, S., Nakonezny, P., Foxwell, A., & Emslie, G. (2019). The development and feasibility outcomes of a youth suicide prevention intensive outpatient program. *Journal of Adolescent Health, 64*(3), 362–369. https://doi.org/10.1016/j.jadohealth.2018.09.015

Larzelere, R. E., Daly, D. L., Davis, J. L., Chmelka, M. B., & Handwerk, M. L. (2004). Outcome evaluation of Girls and Boys Town's family home program. *Education and Treatment of Children, 27*(2), 130–149.

Leon, S. C., Jhe Bai, G., Fuller, A. K., & Busching, M. (2016). Emergency shelter care utilization in child welfare: Who goes to shelter care? How long do they stay? *American Journal of Orthopsychiatry, 86*(1), 49–60. https://doi.org/10.1037/ort0000102

Lewin, A. B., Storch, E. A., Merlo, L. J., Adkins, J. W., Murphy, T., & Geffken, G. A. (2005). Intensive cognitive behavioral therapy for pediatric obsessive compulsive disorder: A treatment protocol for mental health providers. *Psychological Services, 2*(2), 91–104. https://doi.org/10.1037/1541-1559.2.2.91

Negreiros, J., Selles, R. R., Lin, S., Belschner, L., & Stewart, S. E. (2019). Cognitive-behavioral therapy booster treatment in pediatric obsessive-compulsive disorder: A utilization assessment pilot study. *Annuals of Clinical Psychiatry, 31*(3), 179–191.

Nock, M. K., & Ferriter, C. (2005). Parent management of attendance and adherence in child and adolescent therapy: A conceptual and empirical review. *Clinical Child and Family Psychology Review, 8*(2), 149–166. https://doi.org/10.1007/s10567-005-4753-0

Ofonedu, M. E., Belcher, H. M. E., Budhathoki, C., & Gross, D. A. (2017). Understanding barriers to initial treatment engagement among underserved families seeking mental health services. *Journal of Child and Family Studies, 26*(3), 863–876. https://doi.org/10.1007/s10826-016-0603-6

Osgood-Hynes, D., Riemann, B., & Björgvinsson, T. (2003). Short-term residential treatment for obsessive-compulsive disorder. *Brief Treatment and Crisis Intervention, 3*(4), 413–435. https://doi.org/10.1093/brief-treatment/mhg028

Pellerin, K. A., Costa, N. M., Weems, C. F., & Dalton, R. F. (2010). An examination of treatment completers and non-completers at a child and adolescent community mental health clinic. *Community Mental Health Journal, 46*(3), 273–281. https://doi.org/10.1007/s10597-009-9285-5

Prescriber's Digital Reference. (2020). *Prescriber's digital reference.* https://www.pdr.net
Reardon, T., Harvey, K., Baranowska, M., O'Brien, D., Smith, L., & Creswell, C. (2017). What do parents perceive are the barriers and facilitators to accessing psychological treatment for mental health problems in children and adolescents? A systematic review of qualitative and quantitative studies. *European Child & Adolescent Psychiatry, 26*(6), 623–647. https://doi.org/10.1007/s00787-016-0930-6
Reed, P., Osborne, L. A., & Corness, M. (2007). Brief report: Relative effectiveness of different home-based behavioral approaches to early teaching intervention. *Journal of Autism and Developmental Disorders, 37*(9), 1815–1821. https://doi.org/10.1007/s10803-006-0306-8
Rice, B. J., Woolston, J., Stewart, E., Kerker, B. D., & Horwitz, S. M. (2002). Differences in younger, middle, and older children admitted to child psychiatric inpatient services. *Child Psychiatry and Human Development, 32*(4), 241–261. https://doi.org/10.1023/A:1015244626238
Ritschel, L. A., Cheavens, J. S., & Nelson, J. (2012). Dialectical behavior therapy in an intensive outpatient program with a mixed-diagnostic sample: DBT in an intensive outpatient program. *Journal of Clinical Psychology, 68*(3), 221–235. https://doi.org/10.1002/jclp.20863
Rudowitz, R., & Garfield, R. (2019). 10 things to know about Medicaid: Setting the facts straight. https://www.kff.org/medicaid/issue-brief/
Salloum, A., Johnco, C., Lewin, A. B., McBride, N. M., & Storch, E. A. (2016). Barriers to access and participation in community mental health treatment for anxious children. *Journal of Affective Disorders, 196,* 54–61. https://doi.org/10.1016/j.jad.2016.02.026
Schlup, B., Munsch, S., Meyer, A. H., Margraf, J., & Wilhelm, F. H. (2009). The efficacy of a short version of a cognitive-behavioral treatment followed by booster sessions for binge eating disorder. *Behavioral Research and Therapy, 47*(7), 628–635. https://doi.org/10.1016/j.brat.2009.04.003
Sherman, M. L., Barnum, D. D., Nyberg, E., & Buhman-Wiggs, A. (2008). Predictors of preintake attrition in a rural community mental health center. *Psychological Services, 5*(4), 332–340. https://doi.org/10.1037/a0013851
Spielberger, J., Scannell, M., & Harden, A. (2010). *Characteristics and outcomes of children served by the Boys Town South Florida family centered services program, 2004–2009.* Chapin Hall at the University of Chicago.
Stancin, T., & Perrin, E. C. (2014). Psychologists and pediatricians: Opportunities for collaboration in primary care. *American Psychologist, 69*(4), 332–343. https://doi.org/10.1037/a0036046
Stein, R. E. K., Horwitz, S. M., Storfer-Isser, A., Heneghan, A., Olson, L., & Hoagwood, K. E. (2008). Do pediatricians think they are responsible for identification and management of child mental health problems? Results of the AAO Periodic Survey. *Ambulatory Pediatrics, 8*(1), 11–17. https://doi.org/10.1016/j.ambp.2007.10.006
Strijker, J., Knorth, E. J., & Knot-Dickscheit, J. (2008). Placement history of foster children: A study of placement history and outcomes in long-term family foster care. *Child Welfare, 87,* 107.
Swift, J. K., & Callahan, J. L. (2010). A delay discounting model of psychotherapy termination. *International Journal of Behavioral Consultation and Therapy, 5*(3–4), 278–293. http://dx.doi.org/10.1037/h0100889

Swift, J. K., Whipple, J. L., & Sandberg, P. (2012). A prediction of initial appointment attendance and initial outcome expectations. *Psychotherapy, 49*(4), 549–556. https://doi.org/10.1037/a0029441

U.S. Department of Health and Human Services. (2020). *2020 Federal poverty levels/Guidelines and how they determine Medicaid eligibility.* Retrieved June 1, 2020, from https://www.medicaidplanningassistance.org/federal-poverty-guidelines/

Weisz, J. R., & Kazdin, A. E. (2018). The present and future of evidence-based psychotherapies for children and adolescents. In J. R. Weisz & A. E. Kazdin (Eds.), *Evidence-based psychotherapies for children and adolescents* (pp. 577–595). Guilford Press.

Wolk, C. B., Kendall, P. C., & Beidas, R. S. (2015). Cognitive-behavioral therapy for child anxiety confers long-term protection from suicidality. *Journal of the American Academy of Child & Adolescent Psychiatry, 54*(3), 175–179. https://doi.org/10.1016/j.jaac.2014.12.004

APPENDIX

Quick Resources, Worksheets, and Handouts

5.1 Diaphragmatic Breathing Script
5.2 Progressive Muscle Relaxation Script
5.3 Guided Imagery Script
6.1 Initial Activity Monitoring Form
6.2 Cognitive Distortions and Examples in Children and Adolescents
6.3 Parent Overview of Behavioral Activation Strategies and Tips
6.4 Parent Resource for Cognitive Restructuring Tips
7.1 Parent Handout on Exposure Therapy
7.2 Sample Fear Hierarchies
8.1 Behavioral Tracking and Intervention Apps
8.2 Mindfulness and Relaxation-Based Apps
8.3 Therapy/Self-Help Apps

QUICK RESOURCE 5.1 — DIAPHRAGMATIC BREATHING SCRIPT

Today we are going to learn about diaphragmatic breathing. Most people engage their diaphragm when yawning or hiccupping. The sensations when engaging the diaphragm are similar to that of yawning and pulling in a sustained breath. The act of yawning forces deep intake and outlet of air. Diaphragmatic breathing, though, does not have to be sparked by something spontaneous like a yawn; it can be learned.

One of the easiest ways to learn how to breathe with your diaphragm is to lie on a flat surface (couch, floor) with a pillow under your head with knees bent (a pillow can be placed under the knees for comfort, if desired). Next, put one hand flat on your chest and put something small, flat, and light (cellphone, playing card, pencil, or other hand) on your stomach, right below the ribcage. Now, focus on breathing in through your nose and pushing your stomach out against your hand. The hand on your chest should remain as still as possible. Once you have taken in a full breath through your nose, breathe out through your mouth, and your stomach should fall inward toward where it started. Again, the hand on your chest should remain as still as possible. As you breathe in and out you should be able to see and feel your stomach rising and falling. The small item on your stomach will help you see this movement more easily. At first when you practice this you will need to concentrate to ensure use of the diaphragm, and you will likely get tired. As you practice more, diaphragmatic breathing will become more automatic and easier. Even just 5 minutes per day can be helpful in developing the diaphragmatic breathing skill.

QUICK RESOURCE 5.2—PROGRESSIVE MUSCLE RELAXATION SCRIPT

To start, focus on your breath and become aware of your own body. Concentrate on being more in tune with the present while also paying attention to your breathing. Once you are appropriately focused, you begin the process of tightening and loosening of muscle groups. In this exercise, you start with your head and work your way to your feet. First, scrunch up your whole face; squeeze your eyes closed, scrunch your nose, and wrinkle your forehead. Notice how your face feels when it is tense. Squeeze a little more. Feel the tension in your cheeks and eyes. Now, relax. Let your face droop down and be completely at ease. Notice how much better it feels to be relaxed than tense.

Next, pull your shoulders up to cover your neck. Pretend you are a turtle pulling your head into your shell. Feel how tight your neck is and how uncomfortable it is. See if you can tense your shoulders any more. Pay attention to how tense your neck and shoulders are. Now, release. Notice how much better it feels to be relaxed than tense. Zero in on the two states and really compare and recognize how it feels to be tense versus relaxed. Now, squeeze your hands. Pretend you have a lemon in your hand and you are trying to squeeze all the juice out. Notice how your forearm and hand feel when they are tense. Keep squeezing; try to get all the juice out. Now drop the lemon and relax your hands and arms. Notice how much better it feels to be relaxed than tense. Compare how it feels to be tense versus relaxed.

To continue this process, one would move onto the stomach, then buttocks, then thighs, then feet, each step along the way ensuring the focus is first on the tension and second on the relaxation. At the end, it is helpful to relax the entire body, as if you were a ragdoll that had no bones or muscles. Then compare that relaxed feeling to how you felt when you first started the exercise.

QUICK RESOURCE 5.3—GUIDED IMAGERY SCRIPT

It is helpful to begin by centering yourself in the moment and in your own body. After this, focusing on your breath by doing 2 to 3 minutes of diaphragmatic breathing is helpful. Finally, bring into awareness a place where you feel safe, relaxed, and comfortable. Imagine all the things you can see, smell, hear, taste, or touch in that space. Really focus on all the elements in that place while continuing to engage in diaphragmatic breathing. A lot of people use a place outside—the forest, the beach, or an open clearing.

If I were to use the beach as my place to focus on, I might describe seeing the ocean and waves, the sand, birds in the distance, crabs crawling on the sand, and the sky. Next, I would describe being able to hear the waves crashing, birds cawing, and maybe children playing somewhere down the beach. I would describe smelling the salt on the wind with the combination of the heat in the air, and feeling the sand and the water on my feet, the wind and ocean spray on my skin. Finally, I would see if there was anything I could taste. Sometimes there is not, but the act of trying to figure it out and fully immersing yourself in that moment is helpful for the exercise. In this case, you might taste salt on the air. When you are ready, come back to the present moment in space and time. Notice how relaxed and at peace you feel.

QUICK RESOURCE 6.1 — INITIAL ACTIVITY MONITORING FORM

Day of the Week: _____

Time	Activity	Like to Do (0–10)	Need to Do (0–10)	Used a Helper (Y or N)
7–8 a.m.				
8–9 a.m.				
9–10 a.m.				
10–11 a.m.				
11 a.m.–Noon				
Noon–1 p.m.				
1–2 p.m.				
2–3 p.m.				
3–4 p.m.				
4–5 p.m.				
5–6 p.m.				
6–7 p.m.				
7–8 p.m.				

QUICK RESOURCE 6.2 — COGNITIVE DISTORTIONS AND EXAMPLES IN CHILDREN AND ADOLESCENTS

- Labeling/Mislabeling
  - Child example: "Eva didn't say 'hey' to me this morning, she's being a meanie!"
  - Adolescent example: "I had to take the ACT twice to be considered for the honors program at the school I'm applying to. I'm not cut out for college."
- Overgeneralization
  - Child example: "I meant to subtract instead of add on question #2 on my quiz. I'm a moron."
  - Adolescent example: "I forgot to open the door for my girlfriend today. I'm a horrible girlfriend."
- Magnification/Catastrophizing
  - Child example: "Mehdi stepped on my new shoes, so now I can never wear them again!"
  - Adolescent example: "I'm grounded for the weekend and can't go out with friends. My social life is over!"
- "Should" Statements
  - Child example: "Javier must pick me as his co-captain because we're best friends. If he doesn't, he's not a good friend."
  - Adolescent example: "I should've been more friendly to Amber before she moved. Now I will never get the chance to apologize."
- Fallacy of Fairness
  - Child example: "Becca shouldn't have gotten to lead the lunch line. She did it last week!"
  - Adolescent example: "Why did Anthony get MVP this season? I scored more touchdowns than he did."
- Fallacy of Change
  - Child example: "Cody wants me to help him win the game, so I'll take the lead."
  - Adolescent example: "Nikita is perfect in every way, but she will feel better if I correct her each time she uses the wrong tense in a sentence."
- Arbitrary Inference/Drawing Conclusions
  - Child example: Walking to the bus stop: "Everyone probably thinks I have cooties."
  - Adolescent example: Sat down next to Juanita in class: "She wishes I chose a different seat."
- Fortune Telling
  - Child example: "My parents want me to invite friends over to play video games. But no one wants to come over and play with me."
  - Adolescent example: "The school dance is soon, and I need to find a date. But I know if I ask her, she's going to say no."

- Jumping to Conclusions/Mind Reading
    - Child example: "The teacher asked us to split into partners, and I choose Requita instead of my best friend Carly because she has an A in the class. Carly must hate me now."
    - Adolescent example: "As I'm walking into class right before the bell rings, everyone is going to stare at my zit."
- All-or-Nothing Thinking/Black-and-White Thinking/Polarized Thinking
    - Child example: "My mom forgot to buy me ice cream! I won't talk to her ever again!"
    - Adolescent example: "Nothing I do will ever make Mr. Pollard think I'm a good student."
- Control Fallacies
    - Child example: "Why should I try to raise my hand in class? He's never going to call on me anyway."
    - Adolescent example: "I can't help the fact I failed my history paper. Mr. Sims knew he shouldn't have assigned that topic to me."
- Personalization
    - Child example: "I'm the reason the entire class got lunch detention because I forgot to ask Mrs. Potts a question."
    - Adolescent example: "I have to stop being friends with Beaux because I'm always the reason he gets into fights."
- Disqualifying the Positive
    - Child example: "Daddy did buy Legos for my birthday, but he really didn't want to."
    - Adolescent example: "He said I was cute, but I know he was just trying to be nice."
- Mental Filter
    - Child example: Teacher usually gives high fives to students as they leave her classroom at the end of the day. "Mrs. Tate didn't give me a high five when the bell rang. She doesn't like me anymore."
    - Adolescent example: Student has never received negative feedback on a presentation: "Why did my teacher yawn at the beginning of my presentation? She's never done that before. I'm going to fail."
- Always Being Right
    - Child example: "My answer was better than Nathan's, but Ms. Ororo gave him the extra-credit point."
    - Adolescent example: "Tori answered Mr. Suarez's question with a perspective different than mine. She wants to prove me wrong. I'm not going to let that happen."
- Emotional Reasoning
    - Child example: "I feel ugly; therefore, everyone thinks I'm ugly too."
    - Adolescent example: "I'm feeling stressed out with all of this homework; therefore, I'm not smart."

QUICK RESOURCE 6.3 — PARENT OVERVIEW OF BEHAVIORAL ACTIVATION STRATEGIES AND TIPS

Why is my child depressed? Distorted thoughts maintain the maladaptive emotions and behaviors you are noticing.

What is behavioral activation? Behavioral activation is a form of behavior therapy that targets the avoidance and withdrawal that cause kids and teenagers to stop participating in previously rewarding activities.

Who is behavioral activation for? It is for children and adolescents who are struggling with anhedonia consistent with depression and those who often avoid behaviors vital to the maintenance of positive mood, commonly seen in individuals with anxiety, depression, and even chronic medical illnesses.

How does behavioral activation work? The child will document current activity involvement during the day and observe the type of unhelpful behaviors they typically engage in, then identify life areas/values/activities that are enjoyable and/or important and engage in those new activities.

Can I help during behavioral activation? Yes! The possibilities are endless. Here are some examples:

- Listen to your child discuss the treatment rationale.
- Periodically monitor the completion of homework associated with treatment.
- Provide feedback to your child and therapist regarding their progress.
- Praise your child when they accomplish tasks, no matter how small, because it's more than they were doing previously.
- Do not do the work for them. Children and adolescents should view you as support rather than the fixer.

Depressed Kid Versus Empowered Kid (Topic: Friendship)

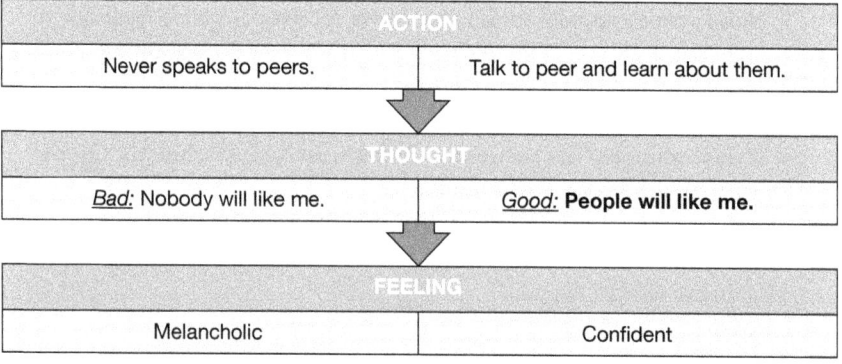

QUICK RESOURCE 6.4 — PARENT RESOURCE FOR COGNITIVE RESTRUCTURING TIPS

What is cognitive restructuring? Cognitive restructuring is a process used within cognitive behavioral therapy to identify negative/irrational thoughts and challenge them with counterevidence in order to ultimately discredit them and improve mood and functioning.

Who is cognitive restructuring for? This practice is beneficial for children and adolescents with a negative outlook on their life, the world around them, and the future, which is commonly seen in those with anxiety and depression.

How does cognitive restructuring work?

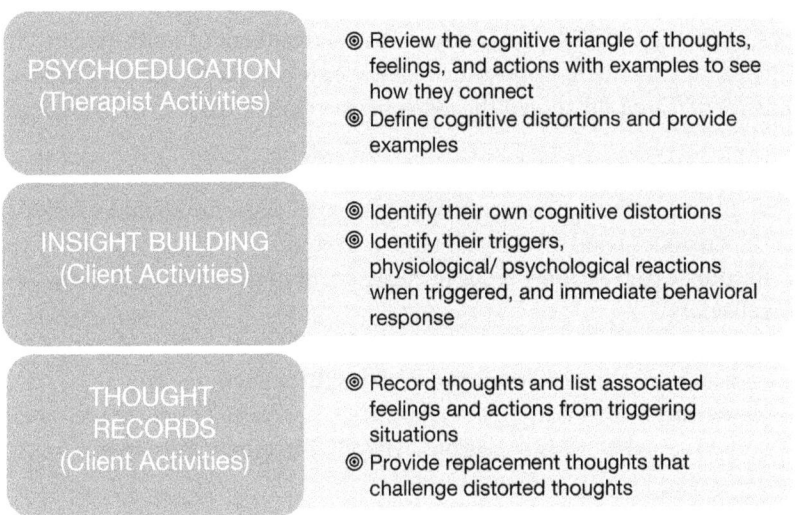

What are some other strategies that strengthen cognitive restructuring? There are many, but here's a few:

- ✓ Socratic questioning: Method that allows the child or adolescent to understand how their mind functions
- ✓ Coping skills: Merger of various strategies that lessen the severity of physiological and psychological distress
    - ❖ Examples: deep breathing, guided imagery, progressive muscle relaxation
- ✓ Checking the facts: Technique that finds evidence to refute distorted thoughts
- ✓ Thought logs: Technique used to identify negative automatic thoughts and then alter them to improved thoughts.

QUICK RESOURCE 7.1 — PARENT HANDOUT ON EXPOSURE THERAPY

Exposure Therapy: A Strategy to Improve Student Anxiety

Dear Parent,

Your student may benefit from a strategy called *exposure therapy*. This handout explains this strategy and how it works. Please call your school's mental health provider (e.g., counselor, school psychologist, social worker) if you would like to learn more.

What Is Exposure Therapy?

Exposure therapy is a first-line, evidence-based treatment of youth anxiety. In exposure therapy, a student works with a counselor to complete exposures and reduce avoidance of feared situations. The following are key exposure therapy strategies:

- **Exposure**—practice of a feared situation
  - Example: For a student afraid of germs, an exposure could be shaking someone's hand or using a public restroom.
- **Response prevention**—reduced engagement in ritualistic and safety behaviors
  - Example: The student afraid of germs could reduce the amount of handwashing and cleaning of surfaces throughout the day.
- **Homework**—the student is given practice exposure and response prevention tasks to complete between sessions, typically with parent assistance

How Does It Work?

- The graph below depicts patterns of anxiety when avoidance is practiced and when exposure therapy is implemented.
- **Avoidance** (jagged line): Anxiety starts high, is temporarily relieved when the feared situation is avoided, but returns even higher when the situation is encountered again.
- **Exposure** (downward-sloping line): Anxiety starts high but gradually decreases through repeated exposure to the feared situation without avoidance.

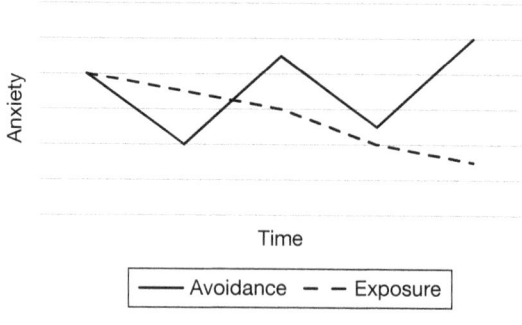

QUICK RESOURCE 7.2 — SAMPLE FEAR HIERARCHIES

Hierarchy for Social Phobia: Presenting in Front of Others

SUDS Rating	Exposure Activity
10 (if needed)	Student presents in auditorium during assembly, with students and teachers present.
9	Student gives 15-minute presentation in front of the entire class.
8	Student gives 5-minute presentation in front of the entire class.
7	Student gives 1-minute presentation in front of the entire class.
6	Student gives 5-minute presentation in front of teacher and small group of students (more critical audience).
5	Student gives 5-minute presentation in front of teacher and three select friendly students.
4	Student gives 1-minute presentation in front of teacher, with no students present.
3	Student raises hand to answer difficult question in class.
2	Student raises hand to answer easy question in class.
1	Student records self-giving presentation and shows it to teacher.
0 (current situation)	Student submits written reports instead of oral presentations.

Hierarchy for School Refusal Exposures: Reintegrating into the Classroom

SUDS Rating	Exposure Activity
10	Student participates in regular schedule for entire school day.
9	Student attends class 7 hours, completes work in office remainder of day.
8	Student attends class 6 hours, completes work in office remainder of day.
7	Student attends class 5 hours, completes work in office remainder of day.
6	Student attends class 4 hours, completes work in office remainder of day.
5	Student attends class 3 hours, completes work in office remainder of day.
4	Student attends class first 2 hours, completes work in office remainder of day.
3	Student attends class first hour, completes work in office remainder of day.
2	Student completes work in nurse's or counselor's office entire school day.
1 (if indicated)	Student completes work in nurse's or counselor's office until lunchtime.
0 (current situation)	Student remains at home during school day.

QUICK RESOURCE 8.1 – BEHAVIORAL TRACKING AND INTERVENTION APPS

Mobile App	Compatibility	Android Manufacturer/Rights Holder	iOS Manufacturer/Rights Holder	Pricing	Description
Daylio	iOS/Android	Habitics	Relaxio	Free; Premium features $2.99/month; $25.99/year	Tracks the user's mood and daily activities.
FLO Period & Ovulation	iOS/Android	FLO HEALTH, INC.	FLO HEALTH, INC.	Free; FLO Premium $9.99/month; $19.99/3 months; $39.99/6 months; $49.99/year	Tracks monthly menstrual cycles.
Habit-bull	iOS/Android	App Holdings	AppForge	Free; $19.99/year	Tracks customizable goals, with a Premium service that expands number of goals.
MapMyFitness	iOS/Android	MapMyFitness, Inc.	Under Armour, Inc.	Free; Premium $5.99/month; $29.99/year	Behavior tracking for exercise.
Medisafe Medication Management	iOS/Android	Medisafe®	Medisafe Inc.	Free; Premium $4.99/month; $39.99/year	Tracks and manages medication regimens.
Moodly: Mood Tracker & Journal	iOS	—	treebetty LLC[2]	Free; One-time upgrade $4.99; Growth bundle $18.99/year; $3.99/month	Tracking app that plots mood and daily activities.

MyFitnessPal	iOS/Android	MyFitnessPal, Inc.	Under Armour, Inc.	Free; $19.99/month; $79.99/year	Tracks nutrition/exercise; allows for customized goals. Additional features include specified training programs and the option to pair with other devices.
One Drop Diabetes	iOS/Android	One Drop	One Drop and Informed Data Systems Inc.	Free; diabetes management equipment through online store	Tracks health behaviors related to diabetes, hypertension, or weight-related concerns.
Productive	iOS/Android	Apalon Apps	IAC Search & Media Technologies Limited	Free; Premium $6.99/month; $11.99/3 months; $29.99/year	Allows user to create and track customizable goals.
Step Younger+	iOS/Android	Keep Walking Health Group[1]	Smillage, Inc.	Free	Pedometer that tracks physical activity.

Note. All app versions are current as of April 2020.

[1]Keep Walking Health Group. (2020). *Step Younger+* (1.6.1) [Mobile Application Software]. Google Play. https://play.google.com/store/apps/details?id=pro.health.steptracker.pedometer.free&hl=en_US

[2]treebetty LLC. (2020). *Moodly: Mood Tracker & Journal* (iOS Version 1.3) [Mobile Application Software]. App store. https://apps.apple.com/us/app/moody-mood-tracker-journal/id1402824590

QUICK RESOURCE 8.2 – MINDFULNESS AND RELAXATION-BASED APPS

Mobile App	Compatibility	Android Manufacturer /Rights Holder	iOS Manufacturer /Rights Holder	Pricing	Description
A Soft Murmur	iOS/Android	Sleepy Rabbit LLC	Polarised Light Ltd.	Free; $1.99 one-time purchase for additional sounds	Sets and blends ambient noises (e.g., rain, fire, crickets) to reduce distress and improve focus.
Calm	iOS/Android	Calm.com, Inc.	Calm.com, Inc.	Free; Premium $14.99/month;$69.99/year; Lifetime subscription $399.99	Guided animations for mindful breathing, sleep stories from various celebrities, and a behavioral tracking feature for mood.
Headspace	iOS/Android	Headspace for Meditation, Mindfulness and Sleep	Headspace Inc.	Free; $12.99/month; $69.99/year	Provides foundational practice in mindfulness through lessons, sleep aids, and exercise routines.
Mindfulness Coach	iOS/Android	U.S. Department of Veterans Affairs[7]	U.S. Department of Veterans Affairs[8]	Free	Provides lessons, goal setting, and a timer for meditating.
Relax and Sleep Well	iOS/Android	Diviniti Publishing Ltd.[1]	Diviniti Publishing Ltd.[2]	Free; $2.99 for individual guided meditations	Meditation app. Offers hypnotherapy and mediation recordings for insomnia, stress, anxiety, mindfulness, sleep, etc.

Spotify	iOS/Android	Spotify Ltd.	Spotify Ltd.	Free; Premium students $4.99; Premium regular $9.99; Spotify for family $29.99 for 5 members; $24.99 for 4 members; $19.99 for 3 members; $14.99 for 2 members. All monthly subscriptions.	Multi-genre music streaming app that offers music, podcasts, and lectures. Also provides mindfulness-based resources (e.g., guided imagery scripts).
Take a Break! Guided Meditation for Stress Relief	iOS/Android	Meditation Oasis[3]	Meditation Oasis[4]	Free; turn off ads $0.99	Provides guided meditations for stress relief and improved sleep.
The Mindfulness App	iOS/Android	MindApps[5]	MindApps[6]	Free; Premium $9.99/month; $59.99/year	Provides foundational practice in mindfulness through lectures, a structured meditation timer, and a guided body scan.
Waking Up: A Meditation Course	iOS	Waking Up LLC	Waking Up LLC	Free; $44.99/3 months; $99.99/year	Provides foundational practice in mindfulness through lectures, a structured meditation timer, and group meditation.

(continued)

QUICK RESOURCE 8.2 CONTINUED

Note: All app versions are current as of April 2020.

[1]Diviniti Publishing Ltd. (2020a). *Relax and Sleep Well* (iOS Version 7.2) [Mobile Application Software]. App store. https://apps.apple.com/us/app/relax-and-sleep-well-hypnosis/id412690467

[2]Diviniti Publishing Ltd. (2020b). *Relax and Sleep Well* (Varies with device) [Mobile Application Software]. Google Play. https://play.google.com/store/apps/details?id=com.imobilize.relaxsleepwell&hl=en_US

[3]Meditation Oasis. (2020a). *Take a Break! Guided Meditation for Stress Relief* (6.8) [Mobile Application Software]. Google Play. https://play.google.com/store/apps/details?id=com.meditationoasis.takeabreak&hl=en_US

[4]Meditation Oasis. (2020b). *Take a Break! Guided Meditation for Stress Relief* (iOS Version 12.1) [Mobile Application Software]. App store. https://apps.apple.com/us/app/take-a-break-meditations-for-stress-relief/id453857236

[5]MindApps. (2020a). *The Mindfulness App* (iOS Version 4.7.91) [Mobile Application Software]. App store. https://apps.apple.com/us/app/the-mindfulness-app/id417071430

[6]MindApps. (2020b). *The Mindfulness App* (Varies with device) [Mobile Application Software]. Google Play. https://play.google.com/store/apps/details?id=se.lichtenstein.mind.en&hl=en_US

[7]U.S. Department of Veterans Affairs. (2020a). *Act Coach* (iOS Version 1.7) [Mobile Application Software]. App store. https://apps.apple.com/us/app/act-coach/id804247934

[8]U.S. Department of Veterans Affairs. (2020b). *Act Coach* (1.1.2) [Mobile Application Software]. Google Play. https://play.google.com/store/apps/details?id=is.vertical.actcoach&hl=en_US

QUICK RESOURCE 8.3 – THERAPY/SELF-HELP APPS

Mobile App	Compatibility	Android Manufacturer /Rights Holder	iOS Manufacturer /Rights Holder	Pricing	Description
Act Coach	iOS/Android	U.S. Department of Veterans Affairs[10]	U.S. Department of Veterans Affairs[11]	Free	Acceptance and Commitment Therapy program used with therapist guidance.
Bloomz	iOS/Android	Bloomz	Bloomz Inc.	Free; Convenience Pack $1.67/month; $19.99/year	Parent–teacher communication app.
CBT-I Coach	iOS/Android	U.S. Department of Veterans Affairs[12]	U.S. Department of Veterans Affairs[13]	Free	Cognitive behavioral therapy for insomnia program used with therapist guidance.
CPT Coach	iOS	U.S. Department of Veterans Affairs[14]	U.S. Department of Veterans Affairs[15]	Free	Cognitive Processing Therapy program used with therapist guidance.
ClassDojo	iOS/Android	ClassDojo	ClassDojo, Inc.	Free; Premium $7.99/month; $39.99/6 months; $59.99/year	Helps educators and parents communicate, set goals, and celebrate student progress.
Dragon Anywhere: Dictate Now	iOS/Android	Nuance Communications, Inc.[3]	Nuance Communications, Inc.[4]	$14.99/month; 149.99/year; negotiated price for groups	Dictation app used for educational or therapeutic interventions.

(*continued*)

QUICK RESOURCE 8.3 CONTINUED

Mobile App	Compatibility	Android Manufacturer /Rights Holder	iOS Manufacturer /Rights Holder	Pricing	Description
First-Then Visual Schedule	iOS	—	Good Karma Applications, Inc	$14.99	Assists parents in providing positive behavior supports for individuals who can benefit from more structure.
Flora	iOS	—	AppFinca Inc.	Free	Gamified productivity timer.
Focus Keeper	iOS	HSM Studio	PIXO Incorporation	Free; Pro version $1.99	Productivity timer.
I Am Sober	iOS/Android	I Am Sober LLC	I Am Sober LLC	Free; Sober Plus $4.99/month; $27.49/6 months; $49.99/year	Tracks sobriety and provides resources to support abstinence.
iReward	iOS	—	Grembe Apps Inc	$2.99	Create star/token charts to reinforce positive behaviors.
Kindle	iOS/Android	Amazon Mobile LLC	Amazon.com, Inc	Free; various in-app media purchases	E-reading program/device that provides access to digital media (e.g., e-books, magazines).
My3	iOS/Android	MHA-NYC	CalMHSA	Free	Safety planning application with emphasis on connecting the individual to an identified support network.

App	Platform	Developer	Publisher	Price	Description
Quit That!	iOS	—	Cozy Apps, LLC[1]	Free; option for donations	Monitors time and financial benefits for abstaining from a habit.
Quizlet	iOS/Android	Quizlet, Inc.	Quizlet, Inc.	Free; Quizlet Plus $1/month; $$11.99/year	Study aid that provides multimodal learning opportunities (e.g., flashcards, games).
Remember the Milk	iOS/Android	Remember The Milk Pty Ltd.[7]	Remember The Milk Pty Ltd.[8]	Free; RTM Pro $39.99/year	Creates reminders and structure for completing tasks (e.g., daily, weekly, monthly, etc.)
Sleep Bug	iOS/Android	Panzertax[5]	Panzertax[6]	Free; Full version $1.99	Ambient noise sound-mixer to improve sleep difficulties.
Sobertool	iOS/Android	SoberTool	Blitzen, LLC	Free; remove ads $3.99	Tracks sobriety and provides resources to support abstinence.
Study Bunny	iOS/Android	Superbyte	Justin Patrick Silang	Free	Gamified productivity timer.
Suicide Safety Plan	iOS/Android	MoodTools	MoodTools	Free	Safety plan application with resources to promote safety behaviors and manage crises.
Tactical Breather	iOS/Android	T2[9]	National Center for Telehealth & Technology[2]	Free	Diaphragmatic breathing resource.
Time Timer	iOS/Android	Time Timer LLC	Time Timer LLC	$2.99	Self-monitor progress with a visual timer.

(*continued*)

QUICK RESOURCE 8.3 CONTINUED

Mobile App	Compatibility	Android Manufacturer /Rights Holder	iOS Manufacturer /Rights Holder	Pricing	Description
YouTube	iOS/Android	Google LLC	Google Inc.	Free; Premium (formerly YouTube Red) $11.99/month; Family $17.99/month; Student $6.99/month	Online video-sharing website that allows users to upload, view, and rate content.

Note: All app versions are current as of April 2020.

[1] Cozy Apps, LLC. (2020). *Quit That!* (iOS Version 2.05) [Mobile Application Software]. App store. https://apps.apple.com/us/app/quit-that-habit-tracker/id909400800

[2] National Center for Telehealth & Technology. (2020). *Tactical Breather* (iOS Version 1.4.3) [Mobile Application Software]. App store. https://apps.apple.com/us/app/tactical-breather/id445893881

[3] Nuance Communications, Inc. (2020a). *Dragon Anywhere: Dictate Now* (iOS Version 1.82) [Mobile Application Software]. App store. https://apps.apple.com/us/app/dragon-anywhere-dictate-now/id1024652126

[4] Nuance Communications, Inc. (2020b). *Dragon Anywhere: Dictate Now* (Varies with device) [Mobile Application Software]. Google Play. https://play.google.com/store/apps/details?id=com.nuance.dragonanywhere&hl=en_US

[5] Panzertax. (2020a). *Sleep Bug* (iOS Version 3.5) [Mobile Application Software]. App store. https://apps.apple.com/us/app/sleep-bug/id467483176

[6] Panzertax. (2020b). *Sleep Bug* (1.6) [Mobile Application Software]. Google Play. https://play.google.com/store/apps/details?id=com.sleepbuginapp&hl=en_US

[7] Remember The Milk Pty Ltd. (2020a). *Remember the Milk* (4.5.5) [Mobile Application Software]. Google Play. https://play.google.com/store/apps/details?id=com.rememberthemilk.MobileRTM&hl=en_US

[8] Remember The Milk Pty Ltd. (2020b). *Remember the Milk* (iOS Version 5.0.18) [Mobile Application Software]. App store. https://apps.apple.com/us/app/remember-the-milk/id293561396

[9] T2. (2020). *Tactical Breather* (1.2.6) [Mobile Application Software]. Google Play. https://play.google.com/store/apps/details?id=t2.tacticalBreather&hl=en_US

[10] U.S. Department of Veterans Affairs. (2020c). *CBT-I Coach* (iOS Version 2.4) [Mobile Application Software]. App store. https://apps.apple.com/us/app/cbt-i-coach/id655918660

[11] U.S. Department of Veterans Affairs. (2020d). *CBT-I Coach* (2.0.3) [Mobile Application Software]. Google Play. https://play.google.com/store/apps/details?id=gov.va.mobilehealth.ncptsd.cbti&hl=en_US

[12] U.S. Department of Veterans Affairs. (2020e). *CPT Coach* (iOS Version 2.4) [Mobile Application Software]. App store. https://apps.apple.com/us/app/cpt-coach/id804271492

[13] U.S. Department of Veterans Affairs. (2020f). *CPT Coach* (1.0.4) [Mobile Application Software]. Google Play. https://play.google.com/store/apps/details?id=gov.va.mobilehealth.ncptsd.cptcoach&hl=en_CA

[14] U.S. Department of Veterans Affairs. (2020g). *Mindfulness Coach* (iOS Version 2.3) [Mobile Application Software]. App store. https://apps.apple.com/us/app/mindfulness-coach/id804284729

[15] U.S. Department of Veterans Affairs. (2020h). *Mindfulness Coach* (2.6.2) [Mobile Application Software]. Google Play. https://play.google.com/store/apps/details?id=gov.va.mobilehealth.ncptsd.mindfulnesscoach&hl=en_US

INDEX

For the benefit of digital users, indexed terms that span two pages (e.g., 52–53) may, on occasion, appear on only one of those pages.

Figures and tables are indicated by *f* and *t* following the page numbers. Numbers followed by n indicate endnotes

AAA (Triple A steps), 56–57
ABC model, 27–28, 28*f*, 32, 37
abuse: mandatory reporting of, 52
Act Coach, 192*t*–94
activity monitoring, 103–4
acute inpatient hospitalization, 174
ADA (Americans with Disabilities Act), 6
ADAAA (Americans with Disabilities Act Amendment Act), 6
adaptive/social skills apps, 152
addiction apps, 151–52
ADDRESSING framework, 73
ADHD. *See* attention-deficit/hyperactivity disorder
Al-Anon, 168–69
all-or-nothing thinking, 14, 185
American Counseling Association (ACA), 49–50, 53–54, 163
American Indian/Alaska Native students, 65, 111–12
American Psychological Association (APA), 27, 49–50, 163
  Ethical Principles of Psychologists and Code of Conduct, 50, 163
  guidelines for recordkeeping, 53
Americans with Disabilities Act (ADA), 6
Americans with Disabilities Act Amendment Act (ADAAA), 6
Android (Android, Inc.) operating systems, 144

anxiety
  Beck Anxiety Inventory (BAI), 31, 105–6
  CBT for, 117, 143–44, 166
  computerized CBT for, 143–44
  intensive treatment of, 173
  questions and phrases helpful in reducing, 126
Anxiety and Depression Association of America Mobile App Clearinghouse, 153
anxiety apps, 153, 154
anxiety disorders
  prevalence of, 1
  sample Tier 2 Counseling Intervention Summary for, 11–19
APA. *See* American Psychological Association
App Store iOS, 144
AppFinca Inc., 152
AppForge Inc., 145–46
Apple Inc., 144
apps (mobile applications), 143–44. *See also specific apps*
  behavioral tracking apps (BTAs), 147–49, 153–55, 189*t*
  communication apps, 152, 192*t*–94
  considerations, 146–52
  diabetes management apps, 147–48, 189*t*

apps (mobile applications) (*cont.*)
    fitness apps, 147–48, 189*t*
    limitations, 152–53
    medication management apps, 147–49, 189*t*
    meditation apps, 149, 189*t*, 190*t*
    mindfulness apps, 149–50, 153–55, 190*t*
    relaxation apps, 149–50, 153–55, 190*t*
    self-help apps, 150–52, 192*t*–94
    sleep hygiene apps, 149, 192*t*–94
    therapeutic benefits of, 144–46
    therapy apps, 150–52, 192*t*–94
    time management apps, 151, 152, 192*t*–94
Aristotle, 151–52
ASD. *See* autism spectrum disorder
assent
    ethical codes, 50–52
    student, 50
assessment measures, 14
attending, 56–57
attention-deficit/hyperactivity disorder (ADHD)
    CBT for, 2–3, 34, 35
    cognitive restructuring for, 107
    empowerment for students with, 85–86
    knowledge building, 84–85
    prevalence of, 1
Audra (case example), 75–76
autism spectrum disorder (ASD)
    CBT counseling for, 34–35
    cognitive restructuring for, 107
autism spectrum disorder (ASD) apps, 148, 152
autogenic relaxation, 90
automatic thoughts, 30, 37, 106–7

BAI (Beck Anxiety Inventory), 31, 105–6
"banana tree" metaphor, 170–71
barriers that interfere with treatment, 167–70
BASC-2 (Behavior Assessment System for Children, Second Edition), 75
BASC-3 (Behavior Assessment System for Children, Third Edition), 105–6
BASC-3 PRS (Behavior Assessment System for Children, Third Edition—Parent Rating Scale), 14

BASC-3 TRS (Behavior Assessment System for Children, Third Edition—Teacher Rating Scale), 14
BATD (Brief Behavioral Activation Treatment for Depression), 101–2
BDI-II (Beck Depression Inventory, Second Edition), 31, 105–6
Beck, Aaron, 25–26, 106–7
    case conceptualization, 36–38
    theories, 30–32
Beck Anxiety Inventory (BAI), 31, 105–6
Beck Depression Inventory, Second Edition (BDI-II), 31, 105–6
Beck Hopelessness Scale (BHS), 105–6
Beck Scale for Suicidal Ideation (SSI), 31
Behavior Assessment System for Children, Second Edition (BASC-2), 75
Behavior Assessment System for Children, Third Edition (BASC-3), 105–6
Behavior Assessment System for Children, Third Edition—Parent Rating Scale (BASC-3 PRS), 14
Behavior Assessment System for Children, Third Edition—Teacher Rating Scale (BASC-3 TRS), 14
behavior problems and disorders
    CBT for, 35
    disruptive behavioral disorders, 1
    intensive treatment of, 173
behavior therapy
    cognitive (*see* cognitive behavioral therapy)
    rational emotive (*see* rational emotive behavior therapy)
behavioral activation, 101–2, 112–13
    limitations, 102–3
    parent handouts, 187
    strategies and tips, 187
behavioral activation hierarchy, 104–5
behavioral intervention technologies (BITs), 143–44
behavioral tracking, 147–49
behavioral tracking apps (BTAs), 147–49, 153–55, 189*t*
behaviorism, 25–26
belly breathing, 90–91
Benson, Herbert, 91
BHS (Beck Hopelessness Scale), 105–6

Index

binge eating disorders, 166
Biopac MP-150 system, 143–44
BITs (behavioral intervention technologies), 143–44
Black identity, 70
Black/African American students, 65, 70
black-and-white thinking. *See* all-or-nothing thinking
Blitzen, LLC, 151–52
Bloomz, 151, 192*t*–94
Bloomz Inc., 151
body language, supportive, 57
booster sessions, 165–66
Bordin, Edward, 60
breathing
 belly, 90–91
 controlled, 91
 deep, 90–91
 diaphragmatic, 90–91, 182
Bresler, David, 93
bridging statements, 109
Brief Behavioral Activation Treatment for Depression (BATD), 101–2
Brief Inventory for Executive Functioning, Second Edition (BRIEF-2), 105–6
BTAs. *See* behavioral tracking apps

Calm (app), 149, 150, 190*t*
Calm.com, Inc., 149
catastrophizing, 14, 15–16, 28, 184
Catholic Charities, 168–69
CBCL (Child Behavior Checklist), 92, 105–6
CBT. *See* cognitive behavioral therapy
CBT Coach, 192*t*–94
CBT for Psychosis, 31–32
CBT-I Coach, 192*t*–94
CDI-2 (Children's Depression Inventory, Second Edition), 105–6
Center for Behavioral Intervention Technologies, 153
Center for Technology in Behavioral Science, 153
change: fallacy of, 184
change ruler, 88–89
change talk, 87–88
Check In/Check Out (CICO), 132
"Checking the Facts" technique, 107–8

Chicano identity, 70
Child Behavior Checklist (CBCL), 92, 105–6
child psychotherapy, traditional, 171
Children's Depression Inventory, Second Edition (CDI-2), 105–6
Children's Health Insurance Program (CHIP), 168
Children's Negative Cognitive Errors Questionnaire—Revised (CNCEQ-R), 110
CHIP (Children's Health Insurance Program), 168
Chomsky, Noam, 26
chronic health conditions, 9–11
CICO (Check In/Check Out), 132
class interventions. *See* universal interventions
ClassDojo, 151, 192*t*–94
ClassDojo, Inc., 151
client(s), 67
 observing, 56
 understanding, 72–73
closed-ended questions, 57–58
closure: preparation for, 163–65
CNCEQ-R (Children's Negative Cognitive Errors Questionnaire—Revised), 110
codes of ethics, professional, 49–52
cognitive behavioral therapy (CBT)
 applications, 1–24
 barriers that interfere with, 167–70
 booster sessions, 165–66
 case examples, 37–38
 class or universal (Tier 1), 4*f*, 4–5
 computerized, 143–44
 core components, 101–16, 117–41
 counseling applications, 33–35
 culturally responsive, 66–70
 efficacy, 2–3
 family-based, 166
 general model, 32
 group considerations, 54–55
 historical development of, 25–26
 individual (Tier 3) level, 4*f*, 5–6, 54–55
 intensive treatment, 173–74
 pragmatic factors, 167
 small-group (Tier 2), 4*f*, 5, 83, 132
 terminating, 163–79

cognitive behavioral therapy (CBT) (cont.)
  theories, 26–32
  theory and research, 25–45
  transgender-affirmative (TA-CBT), 75–76
  trauma-focused (TF-CBT), 107, 128, 131–33
  treatment options, 170–75
cognitive distortions
  assessing, 110
  examples, 186
  rating scales for, 110
cognitive restructuring, 106–7, 112–13
  by assessing cognitive distortions, 110
  case study, 111–12
  developmental considerations, 127
  disability considerations, 127
  efficacy, 110–11
  by "evaluating the evidence," 107–8
  with exposure therapy, 126–28
  with guided imagery, 108
  inhibitory learning and, 127–28
  parent handouts, 188
  Socratic method, 109–10
  strategies that strengthen, 187
  techniques commonly applied, 107–10
  time considerations, 127
cognitive skills, 126–27
cognitive therapy (CT), 31
  applications, 31
  characteristic approach, 38
  influence, 31
  mindfulness-based (MBCT), 93–94, 149
  Mindfulness-Based Cognitive Therapy, 93–94
  sequential intervention goals, 31
cognitive triad model, 30f, 30
collaboration, 86
communication apps, 152, 192t–94
compensating strategies, 85f, 85
complex trauma, 131
computerized CBT, 143–44
conduct disorder
  CBT for, 35
  prevalence of, 1
confidentiality
  ethical codes, 50–52
  example statements about, 51–52
conjunctive faith, 69

consent
  ethical codes, 50–52
  NASP Standard I.1.2, Consent to Establish a School Psychologist–Client Relationship, 50–51
  parental, 50
  rule exceptions, 48
control fallacies, 29, 37, 185
controlled breathing, 91
Coping Power Program (CPP), 35, 54
coping/compensating strategies, 85f, 85
counseling
  CBT applications, 33–35
  IDEA categories most amenable for, 8
  legal guidelines, 48–49
  microskills for, 55–59
  preparation for, 47–63
  sample reports, 11–19
  school-based, 11–19
  Tier 2 Counseling Intervention Summary (sample), 11–19
CPP (Coping Power Program), 35
credentialing, 167–68
CT. See cognitive therapy
cultural differences, 71, 75
cultural self-awareness, 72
cultural strengths, 74
culturally relevant challenges, 75
culturally relevant material, 73–74
culturally responsive services, 65–81
culturally responsive therapy, 66–70
  ADDRESSING framework for, 73
  barriers to treatment, 71–75
  individualized treatment, 73–75

Daylio, 145–46, 153–55, 189t
DBT (dialectical behavior therapy), 107–8
deep breathing, 90–91
depression
  computerized CBT for, 143–44
  major, 1
  prevalence of, 1–2
  triad of, 30f, 30
desensitization, systematic, 118
developmental considerations, 67–70, 127
diabetes management apps, 147–48, 189t
Diagnostic and Statistical Manual of Mental Disorders (DSM), 8

Index   205

dialectical behavior therapy (DBT), 107–8
diaphragmatic breathing, 90–91, 182
disability considerations, 127
disordered thinking
  assessing, 110
  examples, 186
  rating scales for, 110
disqualifying the positive, 185
disruptive behavioral disorders, 1
diversity, 65–66, 67–68
Dragon Anywhere: Dictate Now, 192*t*–94
drawing conclusions, 30–31, 184
DSM *(Diagnostic and Statistical Manual of Mental Disorders)*, 8

eating disorders
  CBT for, 166
  intensive treatment of, 173
ED (emotional disturbance), 8–9
electronic or virtual telehealth, 51–52
Ellis, Albert, 25–26
  ABC model, 27–28, 28*f*
  case conceptualization, 36–38
  theories, 27–29
emergency shelter care, 173
emotional disorders, 2
emotional disturbance (ED), 8–9
emotional processing theory (EPT), 118–19
emotional reasoning, 107–8, 185
empathy, 109
Employee Assistance Programs, 164–65
empowerment, 85*f*, 85–86
  encouraging, 58–59
EPT (emotional processing theory), 118–19
Ethical Principles of Psychologists and Code of Conduct (APA), 50, 163
ethics codes, 49–52
ethnic identity, 70
ethnic minorities, 65
  developmental considerations, 70
  related mental health challenges, 67–68, 71
evidence: "evaluating the evidence" technique, 107–8
expectancy violation, 119, 125

exposure(s), 120
  imaginal, 121
  interoceptive, 121
  virtual reality, 121
  in vivo, 120–21, 130–31
exposure and response prevention (E/RP), 3, 143–44
exposure therapy, 117–26
  case report, 133–34
  cognitive restructuring with, 126–28
  cognitive skills during, 126–27
  components, 120–22
  developing fear hierarchies, 123–24
  developmental considerations, 127
  disability considerations, 127
  examples, 125
  homework, 122, 188
  key strategies, 188
  parent handout, 188
  parental involvement, 123
  relapse prevention, 122–23
  sample tasks, 17
  theoretical framework, 118–19
  time considerations, 127
  trauma-focused, 128–33
  treatment progression, 124–26
extended care, 166–67
externalizing problems, 33, 34–35

Face Your Fears intervention, 35
fairness: fallacy of, 75, 184
faith, 69
faith development theory, 69
Family Educational Rights and Privacy Act (FERPA), 48
  overlap with HIPAA, 49
  provisions regarding recordkeeping, 53
family-based CBT
  booster sessions, 166
  in-home family services (IHFS), 168–69, 172–73
fear hierarchy(-ies)
  developing, 123–24
  samples, 188
fear ladders. *See* fear hierarchy(-ies)
fear structures, 118–19
Federal Child Abuse Prevention and Treatment Act (CAPTA), 52

FERPA. *See* Family Educational Rights and Privacy Act
"fight or flight" response, 91
financial considerations, 167–69
First-Then Visual Schedule, 152, 192*t*–94
fitness apps, 147–48, 189*t*
FLO HEALTH, INC., 147–48
Flora, 152, 192*t*–94
Focus Keeper, 152, 192*t*–94
fortune telling, 184
foundational skills, 109–10
Fowler, James, 69
Freud, Sigmund, 25, 143
Friends for Life (FRIENDS) program, 54

gamification, 147
gender development, 68
gestalt therapy, 107
Good Karma Applications, Inc., 152
Grembe Apps Inc., 152
group CBT, 54–55
guided imagery, 93, 108, 183
guided meditation. *See* meditation

Habit-bull, 145–46, 148, 189*t*
habituation, 118
handouts, 181–94
Harris, Sam, 149
Headspace app, 149, 150, 190*t*
Headspace Inc., 149
health information, protected (PHI), 48–49
Health Insurance Portability and Accountability Act (HIPAA), 48–49
  overlap with FERPA, 49
  provisions regarding recordkeeping, 53
the HEALTHY program, 74
Hinduism, 93–94
HIPAA. *See* Health Insurance Portability and Accountability Act
Hispanic students, 65
HIT-Q (How I Think Questionnaire), 110
homework
  behavioral activation hierarchy, 104–5
  exposure therapy, 122, 188
  therapy, 55, 104–5
hopelessness, 105–6

hospitalization
  acute inpatient, 174
  partial hospitalization programs (PHPs), 173
How I Think Questionnaire (HIT-Q), 110

I Am Sober app, 151–52, 192*t*–94
I Am Sober LLC, 151–52
IAC Search & Media Technologies Limited, 148
IAPS (International Affective Picture System), 92
IDEA (Individuals with Disabilities Education Act), 7–8
IDEA Improvement Act, 7
identity
  racial/ethnic, 70
  -related psychological distress, 71
IEPs (individualized education programs), 7–8
IHFS (in-home family services), 168–69, 172–73
illogical beliefs, 37
imagery, guided, 93, 108, 183
imaginal exposure, 121
iMedical Apps, 153
impulse control, 29, 85
in vivo exposure, 120–21, 130
Indigenous American identity, 70
individual interventions (Tier 3), 4*f*, 5–6, 54–55
individualized education programs (IEPs), 7–8
  counseling preparation for, 47
  medication options, 175
individualized treatment, 73–75
Individuals with Disabilities Education Act (IDEA), 7–8
individuative-reflective faith, 69
inferences, arbitrary, 30–31, 184
information processing theory (IPT), 30–31
inhibitory learning, 119, 127–28
in-home family services (IHFS), 168–69, 172–73
Initial Activity Monitoring Form, 184–85
insurance plans, 167–68

Index

intensive outpatient programs (IOPs), 173
intensive treatment, 173–74
internalizing problems, 33–34
International Affective Picture System (IAPS), 92
interoceptive exposure, 121
interpersonal control, 29
interruptions: Triple A steps (AAA) for, 56–57
interventions. *See also specific interventions*
  design and implementation, 14–16
  evaluation and outcome, 16, 17*f*
interviews
  Jones Intentional Multicultural Interview Schedule (JIMIS), 73
  motivational interviewing, 86–89
  student interviews, 14
  teacher interviews, 12–13
IOPs (intensive outpatient programs), 173
IPT (information processing theory), 30–31
iReward, 152, 192*t*–94

Jacobson, Edmund, 92
Jones Intentional Multicultural Interview Schedule (JIMIS), 73, 75
jumping to conclusions, 30–31, 185

Kabat-Zinn, Jon, 93–94
Kahoot!, 147
Kindle, 150, 192*t*–94
knowledge building, 84–85, 85*f*

labeling/mislabeling, 184
language
  change talk, 87–88
  encouraging/paraphrasing/summarizing, 58–59
  open/closed-ended questions, 57–58
  self-talk, 15
  supportive body language, 57
Latinx students, 74
learning, inhibitory, 119, 127–28
learning disorders, 1
legal guidelines, 48–49
LGBTQ+ youth, 66, 69, 71

listening, reflective, 87
logistic considerations, 169

magnification/catastrophizing, 184
maladaptive beliefs, 30–31
mandatory reporting, 52
MapMyFitness, 147–48, 189*t*
MBCT (mindfulness-based cognitive therapy), 93–94, 149
MBSR (mindfulness-based stress reduction), 149
Medicaid, 168
medication management apps, 147–49, 189*t*
medication options, 174–75
Medisafe, 147–49, 189*t*
meditation, 90
meditation apps, 149, 189*t*, 190*t*
mental filters, 185
mental health challenges and disorders, 71
  negative impact of, 2
  prevalence of, 1–2
mental health services
  culturally responsive, 65–81
  delivery of, 2
  Medicaid benefits, 168
  outpatient, 170–71
mHealth app, 143–44
MI (motivational interviewing), 86–89
micro skills, 55–59, 109–10
mind reading, 185
mindfulness, 93–95
mindfulness apps, 149–50, 153–55, 190*t*
Mindfulness Coach, 190*t*
mindfulness-based cognitive therapy (MBCT), 93–94, 149
mindfulness-based stress reduction (MBSR), 149
mobile applications. *See* apps
mobile operating systems (mOS), 144
monitoring activity, 103–4, 105–6, 184–85
mood disorders, 166
Moodly, 189*t*
MoodTools, 151
motivational interviewing (MI), 86–89
multifaceted care, 166–67
multi-racial students, 65

Multi-Tiered Systems of Support (MTSS), 3–6, 4f, 83
  counseling preparation for, 47
  Tier 1 (universal), 4f, 4–5
  Tier 2 (small-group), 4f, 5, 83, 132
  Tier 3 (individual), 4f, 5–6
My 3, 151, 155, 192t–94
MyFitnessPal, 147–48, 189t
mythic-literal faith, 69

Nar-Anon, 168–69
narratives, trauma, 128–30
National Association of School Psychologists (NASP), xiii, 49–51, 145, 163
National Association of Social Workers (NASW), 49–50, 163
National Center for Telehealth and Technology, 153
National Center of Educational Statistics (NCES), 65
negative thinking, 30, 37
negative triad model, 30f, 30
Northwestern University, 153
Number Cancellation Test (NCT), 91

observation(s)
  client observation, 56
  sample, 13
obsessive-compulsive disorder (OCD)
  CBT for, 117, 166
  intensive treatment of, 173
OHI (other health impairment), 9
One Drop Diabetes app, 189t
open-ended questions, 57–58, 109
oppositional defiant disorder (ODD), 33
  CBT for, 35
  prevalence of, 1
other health impairment (OHI), 9
outpatient mental health services, 170–71
overgeneralization, 184

PANAS (Positive and Negative Affect Schedule), 91
paneling, 167–68
paraphrasing, 58–59, 87
parental consent, 50

parents
  handouts for, 187–88
  involvement in exposure therapy, 123
  involvement in TF-CBT, 130
  sample interview with, 13
partial hospitalization programs (PHPs), 173
PASCET (Primary and Secondary Control Enhancement Training), 54
pastoral care, 168–69
perceived challenges, 167, 169–70
perceptual control theory, 27
personalization, 185
perspective taking, 69
PHI (protected health information), 48–49
phobia(s)
  simple, 1
  social, 1, 188
PHPs (partial hospitalization programs), 173
physical impairments, 7
PIXO Inc., 152
PMR (progressive muscle relaxation), 91–92, 182–83
Polarised Light Ltd., 149–50
polarized thinking, 185
polytherapy, 155
positive activities, 131–32
positive affirmations, 85–86
Positive and Negative Affect Schedule (PANAS), 91
positive behavior: ways to reinforce, 152
positive thoughts
  disqualifying, 185
  ways to develop, 74
prayer, 67
preparation
  for closure, 163–65
  for counseling, 47–63
Primary and Secondary Control Enhancement Training (PASCET), 54
primary care pediatric psychology, 170–71
private insurance, 167–68
private pay, 169
probing questions, 109, 110

Index

problem solving
  externalizing problems, 33, 34–35
  problem description and analysis, 12–14
Productive (app), 148, 189t
professional ethics codes, 49–52
progressive muscle relaxation (PMR), 91–92, 182–83
progress-monitoring systems, 105–6
protected health information (PHI), 48–49
psychiatric disorders
  negative impact of, 2
  prevalence of, 1–2
  severe, 174
psychoanalysis, 25
psychoeducation
  key premises, 83–84
  three-phase approach to, 83–86, 85f
psychointegration, 39n.1
psychotherapy
  CBT for Psychosis, 31–32
  primary care pediatric psychology, 170–71
  traditional child psychotherapy, 171
public insurance, 168

questions
  helpful in reducing anxiety, 126
  open/closed-ended, 57–58
  open-ended, 109
  probing, 109, 110
  to prompt finding evidence for and against worried thoughts, 126
  scaling, 106
  Socratic questioning, 109–10
quick resources, 181–94
Quit That!, 192t–94
Quizlet, 150, 192t–94
Quizlet, Inc., 150

racial/ethnic identity, 70
racial/ethnic minorities, 65
  developmental considerations, 70
  related mental health challenges, 67–68, 71
RADS-2 (Reynolds Adolescent Depression Scale- Second Edition), 75
randomized controlled trials (RCTs), 25
rating scales, 105–6, 110

rational emotive behavior therapy (REBT), 27–29, 107
  ABC model, 37
  applications, 29
  case example, 37–38
  characteristic approach, 37–38
  influence, 29
rational-emotive therapy (RET), 27
RCMAS-2 (Revised Children's Manifest Anxiety Scale, Second Edition), 105–6
RCTs (randomized controlled trials), 25
reasoning, emotional, 107–8, 185
REBT. See rational emotive behavior therapy
recordkeeping
  guidelines for, 53–54
  professional, 52–54
referrals, 163–79
  for extended or multifaceted care, 166–67
reflection of feelings, 59, 109, 110
reflective listening, 87
Rehabilitation Act, 6
relapse prevention, 122–23
Relax and Sleep Well app, 190t
relaxation
  autogenic, 90
  progressive muscle (PMR), 91–92, 182–83
relaxation apps, 149–50, 153–55, 190t
relaxation training, 89–93
Relaxio S.R.O., 145–46
religion, 67–68
Remember the Milk app, 192t–94
reports and reporting
  mandatory reporting, 52
  sample school-based counseling report, 11–19
residential programs, 173–74
resources, 181–94
respite care, 173
response prevention, 121–22, 188
RET (rational-emotive therapy), 27
Revised Children's Manifest Anxiety Scale, Second Edition (RCMAS-2), 105–6
Reynolds Adolescent Depression Scale- Second Edition (RADS-2), 75

rightness: always being right, 185
Rossman, Martin, 93

scaling questions, 106
school refusal, 133, 188
SC-TF-CBT (stepped-care TF-CBT), 132–33
Section 504 plans, 6–7
self-awareness, cultural, 72
self-derogatory statements, 13
self-help apps, 150–52, 192*t*–94
self-help groups, 168–69
self-maps, 16
self-talk, 15
separation anxiety, 1
sexuality, 69
shelters, 173
"Should" statements, 14, 15–16, 28, 184
Silang, 152
Sleep Bug, 192*t*–94
sleep hygiene apps, 149, 190*t*, 192*t*–94
Sleep Stories, 149
small-group interventions (Tier 2), 4*f*, 5, 83, 132
smartphones, 144
SoberTool app, 151–52, 192*t*–94
social media, 146–47
social phobia, 1, 188
social skills apps, 152
social supports, 90
Socrates, 109
Socratic questioning, 31, 38, 109–10
A Soft Murmur, 149–50, 190*t*
special education services, 7
specialty care, 171–72
Spiritual Interventions in Child and Adolescent Psychotherapy (Walker and Hathaway), 74
spirituality, 67–68, 104
Spotify, 149–50, 190*t*
SSI (Beck Scale for Suicidal Ideation), 31
Step Younger+ app, 189*t*
stepped-care TF-CBT (SC-TF-CBT), 132–33
stress management, 143–44
stress management apps, 190*t*
Strong Start program, 74

Strong Teens for Latinx students: Jóvenes Fuertes, 74
student assent, 50
Study Bunny, 152, 192*t*–94
Subjective Units of Distress Scale (SUDS), 15
substance abuse
  intensive treatment of, 173
  prevalence of, 1–2
substance abuse apps, 151–52, 192*t*–94
suicidal behavior
  apps for, 151, 192*t*–94
  Beck Scale for Suicidal Ideation (SSI), 31
  intensive treatment of, 173
suicide, 2
Suicide Safety Plan, 151, 192*t*–94
summarizing, 59, 110
supportive body language, 57
synthetic-conventional faith, 69
systematic desensitization, 118

TA-CBT (transgender-affirmative CBT), 75–76
Tactical Breather app, 192*t*–94
Take a Break! app, 190*t*
teacher interviews, 12–13
technology, 143–61
  behavioral intervention technologies (BITs), 143–44
  case study, 153–55
  rationale for incorporating, 143–44
  therapeutic benefits of, 144–46
Teen Alcohol Rehab, 168–69
telehealth, 51–52
terminating therapy, 163–79
TF-CBT. *See* trauma-focused CBT
theory, 25–45
therapeutic alliance, 60
therapy apps, 150–52, 192*t*–94
therapy homework, 55, 104–5, 122
thought records, 108–9
thoughts
  all-or-nothing thinking, 14, 185
  automatic, 30, 37, 106–7
  disordered thinking, 110, 186
  negative thinking, 30, 37
  worried, 126

Tier 1 (universal), 4f, 4–5
Tier 2 (small-group), 4f, 5, 83, 132
Tier 2 Counseling Intervention Summary (sample), 11–19
Tier 3 (individual), 4f, 5–6, 54–55
time considerations, 127
time management apps, 151, 152, 192t–94
Time Timer, LLC, 151
Time Timer app, 151, 192t–94
Tolman, E. C., 26
Tourette syndrome, 9
tracking
  behavioral, 147–49, 153–55, 189t
  verbal, 57
traditional child psychotherapy, 171
training, relaxation, 89–93
transgender youth, 68
transgender-affirmative CBT (TA-CBT), 75–76
transition planning, 164–65
trauma, complex, 131
trauma narratives, 128–30
  cognitive processing of, 129
  parent involvement in, 130
trauma-focused CBT (TF-CBT), 107, 128–33
  implementation considerations, 131–32
  parent involvement, 130

school-specific considerations, 132
stepped-care models, 132–33
treatment barriers, 71–75, 167–70
treatment options, 170–75
Trevor Project, 151
triad of depression, 30f, 30
Triple A steps (AAA), 56–57

United Healthcare, 167–68
universal interventions (Tier 1), 4f, 4–5
universalizing faith, 69

values: identifying, 104
virtual reality, 121, 143–44
virtual telehealth, 51–52

Waking Up: A Meditation Course, 149, 190t
Waking Up LLC, 149
Watson, John B., 25–26
White identity, 70
White students, 65–66
whole-class interventions. *See* universal interventions
Wolpe, Joseph, 93
working alliance, 60
worksheets, 181–94
worried thoughts, 126

www.ingramcontent.com/pod-product-compliance
Ingram Content Group UK Ltd.
Pitfield, Milton Keynes, MK11 3LW, UK
UKHW021329180426
11947UKWH00017B/1527